Han~~dbook~~ ~~of Clinical Nursing Research~~

Jeanette Robertson RN,MSc,GDipInf&LibStud,BSc,DipPhysEd is the Nurse Researcher at the Princess Margaret Hospital for Children, Perth, Western Australia. Before taking up the inaugural position of Nurse Researcher in 1988, she lectured in the undergraduate nursing program at the Western Australian Institute of Technology (now Curtin University). Prior to that she completed her MSc in Nursing Education at Edinburgh University and her midwifery training at King Edward Memorial Hospital for Women.

For all nurses who seek to improve patient care with thanks to Keith, Peter and Gavin who made it possible.

Handbook of Clinical Nursing Research

Edited by

Jeanette Robertson RN MSc(Edin) GDipInf&LibStud(Curtin)
BSc(UWA) Dip Phys Ed(Melb) FRCNA AALIA

CHURCHILL LIVINGSTONE
MELBOURNE EDINBURGH LONDON MADRID NEW YORK AND TOKYO 1994

CHURCHILL LIVINGSTONE
Medical Division of Longman Group UK Limited

Distributed in Australia by Longman Cheshire Pty Limited,
Longman House, Kings Gardens, 95 Coventry Street, South
Melbourne 3205, and by associated companies, branches and
representatives throughout the world.

First edition 1994

National Library of Australia Cataloguing-in-Publication Data

Handbook of clinical nursing research.
  Includes index.
  ISBN 0 443 04866 5.

  1. Nursing—Research—Methodology. 2. Clinical
  medicine—Research—Methodology. I. Robertson, Jeanette,
  1950– .

610.73072

For Churchill Livingstone in Melbourne
Publisher: Judy Waters
Illustrator: Michael Lindell
Editorial: Pam Lewis
Copy Editing: John Macdonald
Desktop Preparation: Sandra Tolra
Typesetting: Alice Graphics
Indexing: Max McMaster
Production Control: Peter Hylands
Design: Churchill Livingstone
Printing: Kuala Lumpur

Preface

As the scope and complexity of nursing care increases, so too does the demand for competent research which substantiates traditional, and validates innovative, practice. With that need in mind, this *Handbook of Clinical Nursing Research* has been compiled to facilitate the conduct of nursing research in the clinical setting.

In keeping with the natural sequence of the research process, Chapters 1 and 2 provide direction for nurses wishing to transform nursing problems into a researchable format and to locate the literature relevant to the chosen topic. Where financial assistance is required to undertake a study, readers will find valuable information in Chapter 3 as to the characteristics of a successful grant application, while in Chapter 4, those issues that can influence an institutional ethics committee's decision to approve a research protocol are discussed—from the perspective of both a committee chairman and a research applicant.

The planning, implementation and ongoing management of clinical nursing research is detailed in Chapter 5. As this type of research seldom runs according to plan however, Chapter 6 has been devoted to a description of the prevention and/or management of common problems associated with the conduct of clinically based studies.

The organisation and processing of quantitative and qualitative data are addressed in Chapters 7 and 8 respectively. Each of these chapters details those aspects of data management, peculiar to each methodology, which facilitate the process of analysis. Finally, as no research can be considered complete until the results are made public, guidance as to the dissemination of research findings through publication, oral presentation and posters is presented in Chapter 9.

Chosen on the basis of their acknowledged expertise in the subject matter of their respective chapters, contributors to the Handbook have emphasised the practical aspects of undertaking research in the clinical setting not generally detailed by other texts. As such the book is intended to complement, rather than compete with, the excellent methodology texts currently available.

Perth, 1994   J.R.

Contributors

Helen Hamilton RN BA (Monash) Dip Soc (LaTrobe) FRCNA
Projects Officer, Royal College of Nursing, Australia

Susan Lutley (nee Bolton), GD Rdg AD Rec (WACAE) AALIA
Faculty Librarian, Health & Human Sciences, Edith Cowan University WA

Sunita McGowan RN BAppSci (WAIT) MAppSc (Curtin) FRCNA.
Co-ordinator Nursing Research, Fremantle Hospital

Pat Rapley, RN BSc (UWA) MAppSc (Nsg) (Curtin) Dip NEd (CNA) FRCNA
Senior Lecturer, School of Nursing, Curtin University of Technology WA

Jeanette Robertson RN MSc (Edin) GDipLib&InfStud (Curtin) BSc (UWA) DipPhysEd (Melb) FRCNA AALIA
Nurse Researcher, Princess Margaret Hospital for Children, Perth, WA

George Sadleir RFD LlB (UWA)
Judge, District Court of Western Australia and Chairman, Research & Ethics Committee, Princess Margaret Hospital for Children

Robin Watts RN PhD (Colorado) MHSc (McMaster) BA (WAIT) Dip NEd (CNA) FRCNA
Associate Professor and Head, School of Nursing, Curtin University of Technology WA

Western Australian Nurse Researchers' Network
Western Australian Nurse Researchers' Network comprises nurses holding designated nurse researcher positions within the WA clinical career structure. Members who contributed to this book were Mary Wilson, Bentley Hospital; Sunita McGowan, Fremantle Hospital; Sue McDonald, King Edward Memorial Hospital; Nadine Gibbons, Mt Henry Hospital; Jeanette Robertson, Princess Margaret Hospital for Children; Trish Furniss, (formerly) Hollywood Repatriation Hospital; Pat Mannion, (formerly) Royal Perth Hospital; Davina Poroch, Anne Williams, Elspeth Oliver, Sue Tudor Owen, and Vera Irurita, Sir Charles Gairdner Hospital; Coralie Hill, Swan District Hospital; and Anne Bartu, Western Australian Alcohol and Drug Authority.

Contents

1. From problem to proposal 1
   Sunita McGowan

2. Searching for information 15
   Susan Lutley

3. Winning finance for your project 31
   Helen Hamilton

4. Satisfying ethics committees 49
   George Sadleir, Jeanette Robertson

5. Planning and conducting research 67
   Western Australian Nurse Researchers' Network

6. Common problems in the clinical setting 105
   Western Australian Nurse Researchers' Network

7. Managing quantitative data 119
   Pat Rapley

8. Managing qualitative data 135
   Robin Watts

9. Disseminating findings 151
   Jeanette Robertson

Resources 171
Books and software

Standards 181

Index 185

1. From problem to proposal

Sunita McGowan

Nursing research has a comparatively short history when compared with other professions. One of the major reasons for this has been the method of nurse training. Until recently most nurses were trained in a hospital setting where service came first and education was a secondary consideration, with the result that nurses had little, if any, preparation in the research process. This is rapidly changing and in many countries nurses, like other health professionals, are educated in colleges and universities. More and more nurses are completing undergraduate and postgraduate courses that provide them with the necessary skills to undertake nursing research.

What is clinical nursing research?

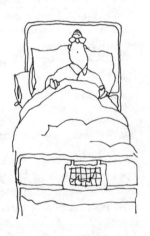

The essence of clinical nursing research has been, and will continue to be, debated by many authors. However, before commencing any research project, it is important to have some understanding of what we mean by nursing research. Wilson (1989) describes nursing research as research into the process of delivering care, and the clinical problems that are encountered in the practice of nursing. There is a popular misconception that research becomes nursing research if it is conducted by a nurse. Research nurses are often employed to facilitate another discipline's research, and as such are valuable members of the team. However, unless this research addresses questions, problems and every day issues that are associated with *nursing* practice, it is not clinical nursing research.

Clinical nursing research addresses questions such as 'Why do we do things this way?' and 'What would happen if we changed a current practice?' It is aimed at investigating nursing problems and generating results that are significant to nursing practice and patient/client outcomes.

Reasons for conducting nursing research

As nurses we are continually confronted with clinical decisions that require choices about approaches to patient care. How do we decide what to do in a given clinical situation? Do we use traditional methods of care, often developed from old wives' tales, intuition, and trial and error situations, do we follow instructions of authority frequently issued by non-nurses, or do we base our judgements on knowledge developed through scientific enquiry? It is sad but true that much of our nursing practice is based upon the former and not the latter.

Increased nursing specialisation

The implementation of career pathways for nurses has been instrumental in recognising and rewarding specialist nursing skills. The recent implementation in Australia of the roles of the Clinical Nurse Specialist and Clinical Nurse Consultant recognises the importance of developing nurses with advanced skills. It is significant that nurses with advanced skills are expected to be able to ask discerning and potentially researchable questions about situations encountered in clinical practice. The increased accountability expected from nurses means that we must examine carefully our clinical practice and ensure that its foundation is research based. We must investigate and substantiate nursing practices that do not have a scientific basis to ensure better patient outcomes and efficient and economical practice. The future of nursing, and in turn nursing practice, is dependent upon research that is designed to generate an up-to-date body of knowledge which can be used to guide our nursing practices.

Justification of current practices

Research generally begins with an unanswered question and it often does not require a large complicated study to answer many of these questions. The following illustrate research questions designed to validate current nursing practice or directly or indirectly improve the outcomes of nursing care.

- Does pressure at the injection site following the administration of subcutaneous heparin minimise bruising at the site?
- Will ice applied to the arm of patients following a brachial cardiac catheterisation reduce the amount of bruising?
- Does the small number of reported blood transfusion reactions warrant the frequency with which patients' vital signs are recorded?
- Which non-invasive interventions (i.e., sitting or standing a patient out of bed, turning on the tap, pouring warm water over the perineal area) assist patients to pass urine post-operatively?

Commonly held assumptions about the value of different nursing practices need to be tested. Many nursing practices are often based on anecdotal remedies and personal preferences with little scientific justification. Lack of scientific evaluation in the past has resulted in many nursing practices, which may have been beneficial, being changed or discarded in favour of new technology. For example, new and improved urinary catheters have made catheterisation a simpler and quicker procedure. Concomitantly, anecdotal evidence suggests that the availability of new generation antibiotics with which to treat catheter induced infections have resulted in a more complacent attitude towards the use of catheters to overcome postoperative micturition difficulties. Until recently the value of simple noninvasive nursing interventions to assist patients experiencing difficulty in voiding, such as sitting or standing a patient out of bed, turning on the tap within the patient's hearing, flushing the toilet, sitting a patient in a warm bath, pouring warm water over the perineal area, have not been tested (McGowan 1992). Better understanding of a problem obtained through research will allow nurses to plan appropriate care for their patients.

Insufficient patient focused research

The perception that nurses can help patients by intuition alone is no more true for nursing than it is for any other health related profession. Research projects that are designed to determine which current nursing practices improve patient care, and whether the implementation of new practices is beneficial to patient care, are needed.

Professional responsibility

If we want nursing to have a major role in influencing the provision of health care, our nursing practices must be shaped by research findings rather than habit. The skills we acquire through college and university education must be used to explore issues that will provide direct recommendations for improving patient care. In a climate of diminishing health care resources we cannot afford *not* to conduct research into the practice of nursing, and not to use the results obtained in improving the cost effectiveness of patient care and defending our professional standards. We need to demonstrate that current and future nursing interventions are economical as well as effective.

Selecting a research topic

The best research problems are usually identified in the clinical setting. Clinical nursing research originates in the workplace and is based on *what nurses perceive are problems*. Every health care setting is replete with possible research questions.

When we move from hospital to hospital there is usually an opportunity to examine traditional nursing practices in different settings and to question their basis. Many inconsistencies are evident in practices and procedures in different hospitals. How many practices are we using without knowing which is the best method or what is the cost differential between different practices? Often the simplest and most common procedures 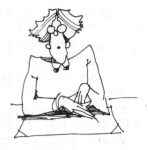 are the ones in need of scrutiny, and it is these procedures that are frequently taken for granted by nurses and so have become part of the rituals of nursing practice.

For example, nurses in different hospitals use a variety of techniques to administer subcutaneous heparin. Although the medical and nursing literature supports the use of a modified subcutaneous injection technique to minimise bruising, until recently there had been little scientific investigation of this practice. In one large hospital where I worked a number of years ago, the practice when administering subcutaneous heparin was to apply two minutes of pressure to the abdominal site post injection to minimise bruising. In another hospital a few kilometres down the road, this practice had grown to five minutes. The only apparent rationale for the difference in practice was if two minutes is good five must be better—not very scientific.

Recent nursing research into this practice indicates that the thigh and arm, in addition to the abdominal site, can be used safely (Stewart & Kinney 1991); aspiration of the syringe has little effect on bruising, and the application of pressure to the site post injection does not reduce the probability of bruising (McGowan & Wood 1990). Another recent study questioned the value of using heparinised saline to flush cannulae in order to maintain patency when intermittent intravenous therapy is used. Two flushing agents, normal saline and heparinised saline, were compared using a paediatric population, and the results demonstrated no significant difference in the incidence of phlebitis or blocked cannulae between the two solutions (Robertson 1992). A further project studied the effect of a modified aseptic technique for the routine care of central venous catheter lines and sites on the incidence of infection. The results revealed that there was no significant change in the rate of central venous catheter line infections when the revised procedure, which cost approximately half that of the previously used procedure, was implemented (Robertson 1991).

Small studies such as these help us to determine *best* nursing practices. Often the therapeutic value of commercial products has never been established. The use of lemon and glycerol solutions for oral hygiene has been a part of nursing practice for well over 50 years. Although used worldwide by nurses in the form of commercially prepared impregnated swab sticks, the ability of lemon and glycerol to clean and moisturise the mouth has never been demonstrated. It has been suggested that the original reason for employing lemon juice in a glycerol solution was related to its potential to stimulate salivary flow (Trenter Roth & Creason 1986).

Nurses working in the oncology area are certainly aware of the detrimental local drying effect of the solution, and laboratory studies cited by Trenter Roth and Creason (1986) have demonstrated that exposure to citric acid (the lemon component) has the capacity to demineralise tooth enamel. Therefore the use of these impregnated swab sticks for oral hygiene seems contraindicated. Nursing research studies that provide direction for clinical practice in maintaining or promoting moisture of the mouth, and cleanliness and comfort of oral tissue surfaces, are still required.

Where to look for a research topic

Currently there is a plethora of nursing practices and task dominated routines that need to be investigated to determine their value and cost effectiveness. Procedure manuals are an ideal place to look for nursing practices for which there is no sound rationale, or basis for the particular procedure. Examine practices that may be based on nursing rituals, old wives' tales or myths, intuition, trial and error, observation or task dominated routines. Colleagues can also often assist by identifying opportunities and promising ideas for research presented by their own work.

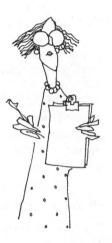

Remember that many procedures regarded as standard nursing practices have *never* been studied scientifically or validated.

Investigate research conducted in an area of practice that interests you. Visit the library and check the nursing journals for research reports that deal with this area of interest. Look for articles that provide opposing points of view or increase your knowledge of the area. Conduct a CD ROM literature search on your topic of interest (see Ch. 2) and ask the librarian where you can locate lists of dissertations or theses, either completed or in progress, which may include your area of interest. Also discuss the problem area with people who have accumulated practical experience in it to obtain their point of view.

Reading journal articles in a speciality area often prompts questions pertinent to nursing practice. Your clinical expertise will allow you to judge whether the research reports you read have included all the variables that could influence the results and whether the reported results are significant for clinical nursing practice. Since research can often pose as many questions as it answers, look for recommendations for future or further research that the author may have suggested.

Often several researchers may identify the same problem as an area deserving further investigation. Suggestions for further research may include the use of additional samples to be studied, other research designs to be used, and new questions to be answered. Remember you do not have to re-invent the wheel, there is a very great need for replication studies to validate the results obtained by other researchers, and to determine if the findings are the same in different settings.

If the environmental temperature could influence a study's results it would be pertinent to replicate the study in a setting with a different climate. For example, results from a hypothetical study conducted in England to assess the ability of various stoma bags to adhere to the skin of patients with a parastomal hernia could not necessarily be applied to patients with parastomal hernias who live in Western Australia. The temperature range in summer in Western Australia, particularly in the North, is very different from that in England and it would therefore be relevant and necessary to replicate such a study in a warmer climate before generalising the results to every patient with a parastomal hernia. Replication studies that support previous research findings strengthen the ability to generalise results to the population from which the study sample was drawn. Bear in mind that established nursing practice should *never* be changed on the basis of a single study's results.

Research questions can also arise as the result of quality assurance or improvement issues or projects. For example, a recent quality assurance study that tested the accuracy of methods used to record hyperthermia in the elderly led a group of nurses to question the reliability and accuracy of infra-red tympanic thermometers.

Defining the problem

It is generally easy to describe a difficult situation, or ponder on a particular problem or question; however, defining the situation or problem so that research can be conducted is usually more complex.

Characteristics of researchable problems

Fuller (1982) identifies a number of characteristics that can assist a novice researcher to determine if a particular problem area is researchable. Firstly the problem should occur in a definable population of patients, secondly the current method of addressing the problem is recognised as unsatisfactory, thirdly the problem must be able to be reliably measured, and fourth any proposed solutions must benefit patient care. A further consideration that I have found useful is the ability for nursing to implement or influence proposed changes.

1. The problem should occur frequently in a definable population of patients.
Before committing yourself to a study you will need to gather information about the size, age structure and other important variables about the population in which the problem occurs. Such data is often available from

routine sources such as the census, morbidity data and infectious disease notifications, etc.

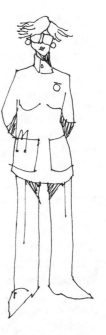

2. The current method of addressing the problem is unsatisfactory to patients and/or nurses.

It is important that you determine if research into the problem is justified by the literature. Maybe there is no satisfactory solution, or little or no evidence to suggest that the current method is the most appropriate. By exploring the problem you will be enabled to challenge what is perhaps taken for granted and question procedures where there is no evidence that they work. A literature search will locate other studies that have tackled the problem, and an examination of the work of others may help you better define and direct the approach you want to take.

3. There is a valid and reliable way of measuring the problem.

The phenomena of interest must be capable of being accurately and objectively recorded and measured. This is one of the most challenging aspects of the research process. By testing the idea on colleagues and asking for their thoughts on how best to measure or record the problem you are often able to decide on an appropriate method. If you intend using an instrument developed by another researcher, choose one that reports a high level of reliability and validity. Once you have found a suitable instrument, often a wide variety of research questions related to the topic can be developed that you can research using that particular instrument.

4. Proposed solutions will improve patient care.

The aim of clinical nursing research is to improve patient or client outcomes. This can be direct, as in the case of evaluation of a new dressing technique, or indirect, if results can demonstrate a saving in nursing time or money when a different procedure is implemented.

5. Nurses will be able to implement or influence any proposed change.

The success of nursing research projects often depends upon factors external to nursing. Decide what it is you wish to accomplish by conducting the research and remember that it is advisable for nursing to have access to, or some control over, the situation or phenomenon under investigation.

If for example, you wanted to evaluate the difference in wound healing between two alternative treatments ordered by medical staff, it would be necessary to gain the co-operation of the medical staff before you start the project. Without their prior agreement you could find that, regardless of your results, the medical staff are not prepared to change the treatments that they order. If prior agreement cannot be reached then it may well be better to admire the problem from a distance and learn to live with it. Appreciation and understanding of the many potential obstacles will ensure that you do not set yourself up for failure.

Converting the problem into a researchable format

The bright idea is usually the easy part and it is also the first important step in conducting any significant research. However, choosing the right question to ask is frequently far more difficult and often presents problems for the experienced researcher. When you have found a problem that you think is interesting and significant, the literature review in the area will assist you to simplify this process.

Questions of a reflective nature, for example—'Should patients be allowed to administer their own medications while they are in hospital?' or 'Do patients receive enough information on care at discharge?' are not researchable in this format. When proposed questions like these examples produce 'yes' or 'no' answers the problem needs to be redefined to enable the development of suitable researchable questions. Perhaps the real problem relates to determining appropriate criteria for allowing patients' to administer their medications, in which case, the question could be worded as 'What factors influence nurses' decisions to allow patients to administer their own medications while in hospital?' or 'What are the factors responsible for nurses' opposition to patients' administering their own medication while in hospital?' Both of these latter questions will allow the researcher to develop instruments to measure the problem. Often discussing the problem with colleagues at this very early stage will assist you with the process of determining appropriate research questions for the study.

When you have defined your problem look for other studies that have tackled the same or a similar problem. Find out if these studies have already been replicated and consider whether there is a need to repeat the same study in similar or different settings.

At this stage it is important to consider the problem in relation to a *known theory* or a *concept* that supports the *rationale* for conducting the research. When little is known about the variables under consideration the aim of the research is to clarify or develop a concept. When the knowledge base is well developed and the relationship among the variables can be predicted then a theoretical framework can be used to support the basis for the research.

Careful consideration of the type of research questions that you wish to ask is important because a clear understanding of the question assists you in determining whether a qualitative or quantitative research methodology is appropriate. *Qualitative* methodologies are most suitable when you wish to analyse the natural, everyday aspects of a situation. When little or no knowledge is available about a certain phenomenon, in-depth interviewing or participant observation may be the most appropriate way to obtain information. In situations where some knowledge about the phenomena or situation under investigation is evident, quantitative analyses are likely to be more appropriate.

In a *quantitative* study, the choice of research design from the selection of the sample and its size to the method of data analysis also depends largely upon the type of research questions or hypotheses (educated guesses) that you generate.

Research questions are appropriate when there is limited knowledge about the topic or when previous research findings are indeterminate or conflicting. Ensure you focus clearly on the research question(s) and adequately define its scope. Research questions must be carefully stated and all major words or terms used need to be operationally defined. For example, a research question that asks 'Is early discharge for herniorrhaphy patients related to post-operative complications?' will require the researcher to define what is meant by early discharge and post-operative complications.

Where *sufficient knowledge or research findings* are available to predict a possible outcome, the use of non-directional (sometimes called substantive) or directional hypotheses are appropriate. A non-directional hypothesis indicates that a difference is expected—whereas a directional hypothesis also specifies the direction of the difference. For example:

- Non–directional hypothesis: there will be a difference in the degree of bruising at the brachial cardiac catheter insertion site post procedure between patients who receive ice packs and patients who do not.
- Directional hypothesis: patients who have ice packs applied to the brachial cardiac catheter insertion site post procedure will have less bruising than patients who do not (McGowan & Power 1988).

If the researcher is unable to predict a difference in outcome between interventions then a null hypothesis may be appropriate. For example:

- Null hypothesis: there will be no difference between the degree of bruising observed at the brachial cardiac catheter insertion site post procedure between patients who receive ice packs and patients who do not.

Prerequisites of a proposal

Relevance of the topic to practice

Before beginning to write a proposal it is important that you are able to explain clearly the magnitude of the problem and its significance to nursing practice. It is particularly important to be able to indicate the clinical relevance of the problem if you are expecting nurses at the bedside to be involved in implementing procedures, interventions, or data collection.

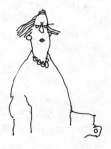

When possible observe the problem first-hand. It is always helpful if you can provide objective evidence of the extent of the problem. This may involve collecting simple statistics, for example, the proportion of patients in a domiciliary nurses' case load with chronic leg ulcers, or the number of patients who complain over a defined period of time of backache after surgery. You may also be able to provide further compelling evidence of the problem, such as photographs of the degree of bruising that can occur following the administration of subcutaneous heparin.

Time frame

Early in the planning process determine the amount of time you will need to complete the study. Since the success of your study is dependent upon the collection of data, particular attention should be spent on the time necessary to collect it. Make sure you check that the subjects you wish to study will be available for recruitment *in sufficient numbers within the time period* set for the study. It is also important to be aware from the very beginning what the approval process for your study is, and approximately how long it will take. The process can extend the intended starting date by three or four months if a number of different committees have to approve the research.

Ensure that you allow adequate time for this process because, if you are asked to make changes or further clarify an aspect of the study, that will also increase the time frame before you can commence the project.

When you have determined an anticipated time frame for the study, if possible allow an additional one to three months (depending upon the size of the study) as a precaution against unavoidable, unexpected problems, which have a habit of occurring at crucial times when research is in progress.

Support infrastructure

Personnel. Determine what infrastructure exists within the organisation to support nursing research. If you intend conducting the research in your own organisation, consider joining a research based interest group if one exists, and where one does not already exist, consider starting one yourself. Valuable information, such as the *practicalities* of conducting clinically based research can be gained when you discuss research plans with colleagues, and frequently support and assistance can be obtained from others who are also undertaking research. Where there is a nurse with specific responsibilities for nursing research contact her early in the planning stage. This will enable you to discuss the feasibility of conducting the study in a chosen setting and allow you to discuss requirements for obtaining permission to conduct the study.

Physical resources. Decide what other resources will be necessary to ensure successful completion of the study. For example, will you need someone to assist with data collection, and will you need access to a computer data base or a statistical software package? Be sure you determine at an early stage in the planning process whether the resources you need will be readily available to you. If a small amount of data is to be collected for routine statistical analyses an electronic calculator may be sufficient, however if you are planning to collect a large amount of data that will require sophisticated analyses, you will need to plan for computerisation early in the research process. One of the first steps in computerising a research project is to design appropriate data collection forms, which allow entry of data from the form into the computer (see Ch. 7).

Research can sometimes be surprisingly expensive and where no funds are available within the organisation to assist with the cost of resources you may need to approach funding agencies or other nursing organisations for assistance (see Ch. 3). Some organisations may be able to provide photocopying, telephone calls, or access to computers, particularly if the results of your study are likely to have relevance in the clinical practice areas and management is supportive of the aims of your study. However, do not assume that assistance will be readily available. Determine what help you can expect before you prepare your proposal and this will avoid disappointment (or panic) at a later stage when you discover that the necessary resources are unavailable.

Enlisting assistance

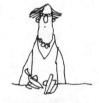

If you require input or assistance from nursing staff to implement your study successfully do not assume that staff will be available, or co-operative, with their time. If it is necessary for you to conduct training sessions for staff that cannot be accommodated within the usual working day (anything longer than 10 minutes is generally prohibitive) determine early in the planning stage whether staff will be prepared to attend sessions in their own time. A circular, giving a brief description of the planned study and asking for expressions of interest to be involved, will give you some idea about the possible level of commitment from staff in the area.

Determine whom you need to obtain *permission* from before you send the circular. If it is at all possible a visit to the area to explain what level of involvement you require, and why, will also improve your chances of staff agreeing to participate. Determine when is most suitable for the staff, and make yourself available at these times. If you need to conduct training sessions, remember that staff will be more likely to attend in their own time if they share your belief about the importance of the planned study, and if the sessions are arranged immediately before or after a rostered shift. It is likely that you will need to be available at meal times for staff who are working permanent night shifts and during the weekend for staff who work only at these times. Where teaching sessions require 30 minutes or more of staff time, the provision of light refreshments or the inclusion of other small 'rewards', such as chocolate frogs, etc., is likely to provide an atmosphere more conducive to learning. Such actions show staff that you appreciate the fact they are prepared to give up their own time to assist with your study. It may also improve attendance ratings at subsequent sessions.

Remember to anticipate the effect of your project on other health professionals. If a change in nursing practice is likely to provoke comment from others, be pro-active and notify them of your project before you commence. Always inform medical and allied health staff if you foresee that any misunderstanding has the potential to hamper your project. A letter which briefly explains the aims and purpose of the project, along with reassurance that it will not impact on medical or allied health practices, will not only avoid potential misunderstanding but also promote the worth of your project. Remember to include an address or phone number where you can be contacted for more information, along with information on the approval you have obtained to conduct the study.

Knowledge base

Be sure that your planned study is within your range of capabilities and recognise your own limitations. You should already know, or be prepared to learn, the skills that will be needed to complete the project successfully. Because more than one skill is likely to be required, it is sensible to be competent in the major skill at least and have some knowledge of the other skills required. If you have had little or no experience with computers, and plan to use a computer, make sure you complete a short course, or gain some basic experience *before* you commence the project. Where you lack major management or research skills required to embark on the project on your own, consider a collaborative study with someone who has the expertise you need.

Determining the appropriate data analysis procedure can be a difficult area, and for this reason some inexperienced researchers leave this until the research proposal is almost complete, or, in extreme situations, until the data has actually been collected. This is not advisable because the method of data analysis is integrally linked to the research design and the selection of the sample size. Inadequate sample sizes are responsible for many a study's inability to produce a statistically significant result. If you do not have appropriate statistical or data analysis skills, it is vitally important that you approach either a biostatistician or someone with this knowledge early in the design phase of the project. Where assistance with data analysis will be required, and you do not have a budget to pay for this, consider negotiating with an experienced researcher or biostatistician for their service in return for co-authorship of reports and publications.

Conclusion

This introductory chapter has discussed briefly a number of aspects that need to be carefully thought about before preparing a research proposal. Many of these aspects are dealt with in greater depth in subsequent chapters. Nevertheless, to ensure that you really are fully prepared for the task of proposal writing, consider the following points before you put pen to paper:

- Can you adequately define the problem and its relevance to nursing practice?
- Do you have your facts right, and will you be able to put forward a sound argument based on the knowledge you have obtained?
- Is the planned project manageable with the available resources and the time span available?
- Will the topic sustain your interest for the length of time necessary to complete the project? Remember even small projects require considerable time and effort.
- Have you considered all the variables that are likely to influence the results?
- Do you know how you will analyse your data once you have collected it?

When writing, ensure that your research proposal describes clearly and concisely what you plan to accomplish. Ensure clarity of thought is evident at all stages in the process. Finally, try not to despair. Remember research takes time and the background work is likely to extend much further than you initially thought it would.

REFERENCES

Fuller E O 1982 Selecting a clinical problem for research. Image 14:60–61
McGowan S 1992 Post operative micturition: a study of difficulties with return of bladder function and the use of nursing interventions. Unpublished Masters thesis, Curtin University of Technology, Perth
McGowan S, Power J 1988 Effect of ice on bruising at cardiac catheter insertion sites (brachial approach). Australian Journal of Advanced Nursing 5(2):27–32
McGowan S, Wood A 1990 Administering heparin subcutaneously: an evaluation of techniques used and bruising at the injection site. Australian Journal of Advanced Nursing 7(2):30–39
Robertson J 1991 Changing central venous catheter lines: evaluation of a modification to clinical practice. Journal of Paediatric Oncology Nursing 8(4):173–179
Robertson J 1992 Intermittent IV therapy: a comparison of two flushing solutions. Unpublished research, Princess Margaret Hospital for Children, Perth WA
Stewart P S, Kinney M R 1991 The abdomen, thigh and arm as sites for subcutaneous heparin injections. Nursing Research 40(4):204–207
Trenter Roth P, Creason N S 1986 Nurse administered oral hygiene: is there a scientific basis? Journal of Advanced Nursing 11:323–331
Wilson H S 1989 Research in nursing, 2nd edn. Addison-Wesley, Redwood City, California, p 27

2. Searching for information

Susan Lutley

Once you have selected a research topic and begun to formulate research questions, the literature review is the next important step. This involves searching, selecting and organising relevant current literature for review to be 'updated, revised and revisited' (O'Connor 1992) throughout your project, particularly as findings in clinical and ethical research change rapidly. You may be apprehensive, not only about the importance of this component of your research, but also about your ability to carry out this task effectively and efficiently. By developing an understanding of *why* the literature search is vital and *how* the literature is organised, combined with adequate planning, will make the process not only less stressful, but it will also certainly contribute to more satisfying and rewarding research and more effective use of time.

Aim of a literature review

The primary purpose of reviewing relevant literature is to gain a broad background knowledge or understanding of the information that is available related to the research problem of interest (Burns 1987). It is important to review relevant literature to assist in securing a starting point or focus for your project, perhaps by identifying the knowledge gaps in the area. The purpose and the timing of the review will also be influenced by the type of research you are conducting.

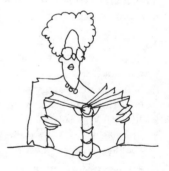

For example, in *quantitative* research it is essential to search the literature at the beginning of the research process. The information located then will normally assist you to clarify the research topic, verify the significance of the research problem, identify relevant studies and theories, select a research design, identify instruments and interpret findings. In this type of research, the search will commonly continue throughout the planning phase of the study—as you refine the research plan and proposal.

The timing and purpose of the literature searching for ethnographic and historical research is similar to that described for quantitative research. In most *qualitative* research, however, it is common for the literature to be reviewed after the data collection. This is particularly true in phenomenological research where researchers run the risk of being influenced by other studies. Similarly, in grounded theory research, only minimal searching of the literature is necessary prior to data collection. Here the main purpose is to combine the literature review with your study findings to determine current knowledge of a phenomenon or to assist in defining concepts and to verify relationships in theory development from the empirical data (Burns 1987).

The literature review itself, as with other steps in research, is a problem solving exercise involving a series of choices: where to look; what to look for; what to select; when to search. It is likely that nurses, who regularly make decisions about patient care, already have the skills to undertake this aspect of the research process. It will greatly assist, of course, if you are also well informed, know some of the pitfalls and some of the shortcomings of searching, and know when and how to obtain additional help. Being aware of the need for a literature review, and having the ability to make appropriate decisions related to your search, will contribute immensely to an effective search strategy.

Basic principles of searching

These are basic strategies that will guide you in identifying and locating relevant sources and so provide the basis for an effective literature review.

1. Plan your search. In this phase you will need to identify the problem, clarify the research topic and define any limitations or special considerations associated with solving the problem (Shockley 1988). While your strategy must be systematic, it should be flexible enough to enable you to make judgements throughout the search.
2. Identify the information sources needed to solve the problem. This involves stating the known sources of information and then searching the literature to identify unknown sources of information. This requires the use of printed indexes, and electronic databases or a combination of both.
3. Select, locate, appraise and organise the articles.

Planning your search

Refining the search topic

To identify your problem, it is helpful to state it clearly in a sentence or two, as simply as possible e.g. To explore the relationship between the healing process and the experiences of pain and sleep in the elderly patient undergoing surgery. Once you have expressed the problem, clarify the subject area by identifying the key concepts, e.g. pain, sleep, surgery, elderly.

Finally consider alternative terms or synonyms for your key concepts, e.g. sleep—insomnia—bed rest; surgery—postoperative care—preoperative care.

Finding facts fast—dictionaries, directories and thesauruses

These reference tools can assist with background information and refine your problem statement. Some useful dictionaries include, *Encyclopedia and Dictionary of Nursing and Allied Health*, *Dorland's Illustrated Medical Dictionary* and *A Dictionary of Nursing Theory and Research*.

Directories such as the *Directory of Nursing Research in Australia*, published by the Royal College of Nursing, Australia, may assist in identifying topics of local research and known researchers with an interest in your area of study.

Many other directories, such as the *World of Learning* will provide useful addresses if you are wanting to contact an institution or individual.

A thesaurus will help you to quickly translate your topic and to identify keywords, sub-headings and relationships between words. The most useful thesaurus is the National Library of Medicine's *Medical Subject Headings* (known as MeSH). The subject headings lists, based on MeSH, related directly to nursing include the lists in the *Cumulative Index to Nursing and Allied Health Literature* (CINAHL) and the *International Nursing Index* (INI). Other similar aids will be discussed in relation to electronic searching. It is important to note that the vocabulary is very controlled (more noticeable when searching printed indexes than with electronic searching, which has the advantage of text searching) and may change as the profession develops and changes.

For example, the term 'critical path' was introduced to CINAHL in 1992 (prior to that you needed to use the broader term 'quality assurance', also used in MeSH). Similarly, the term 'clinical indicators' was introduced in 1992 as a more specific term than 'patient care plans'.

Note also that terms like 'caring', 'nursing care plans' and 'qualitative studies' are used in the nursing subject lists and not in MeSH. Be aware too that American spelling is used throughout these lists, e.g. pediatrics, gynecology, etc.

Defining the span of your search

Special considerations during the planning of a search strategy may include consulting the literature of other disciplines, defining time limits or geographic or age group restrictions. Depending on your selected topic and the type of research, it may be necessary to broaden your search to other discipline areas. Many studies may require you to search literature in areas including psychology, medicine and education. For example, the psychology literature may be useful for our sample topic related to sleep. Also, if your research is qualitative, the empirical information is frequently obtained from literature in related fields, as this type of methodology is relatively new in nursing (Burns 1987). These factors will, in turn, determine which printed indexes and databases you will need to search.

Time factors will also require consideration during planning. Not only will you need to determine when you should conduct the search, but also how long it should take. The latter is often underestimated, as the process usually takes approximately 10% of the total research time.

It will also be helpful to define the time span of the search before you begin; many years may need to be searched to obtain comprehensive coverage. For clinically based problems (which are often the subject of constant review), it is recommended that you begin by searching the most recent indexes and work backwards until the information becomes too out of date.

Finally you will need to decide on the coverage of the literature. For example, do you need to limit the scope to Australia; to just the English language, or to a particular age group? These decisions, made early in your planning, will assist in identifying useful, current sources of information.

Organisation of the nursing literature

The literature for nursing, as for other professions, exists in printed form or computer based form. Within either of these forms, it can be divided into primary literature, informal literature (such as unpublished reports) and secondary literature.

Primary sources vs secondary sources. Your own research will become a primary source of information and, when published, will contribute to the primary literature. Your review of the literature should be mainly primary sources, consisting of journal articles, published conference papers and books. Secondary sources consist mostly of indexes and abstracts, and will assist you in identifying primary literature.

Empirical and theoretical information. There are some types of literature which are best not included in the literature review. While the anecdotes, case studies, letters and commentaries you locate in the searching of your topic may be of interest, these subjective sources are not generally known for their scientific rigour and are therefore best omitted from your review, which should consist primarily of empirical and theoretical information.

Empirical information is generated from previous studies conducted on the selected or related research problem (Burns 1987) and may include research based published articles or unpublished studies such as theses. The theoretical and conceptual type of information may require a search related to particular nursing theorists. Planning your needs and considering these factors will assist you in limiting your searching to relevant and valid research studies and theoretical articles.

Identifying the information sources

It is crucial to the success of your study that you explore all known sources of information. This may include consulting a known expert, a fellow researcher, or may include reviewing a known published article or chapter from a book.

Known expert

It is very sensible to contact persons or organisations familiar with your topic. It can save you a lot of time and lead to many relevant sources of information.

Nurses are more and more prepared and encouraged to share research work at conferences or seminars and by publishing in newsletters and research journals.

Known studies

It is quite probable your interest in a research topic originated not only from a clinical issue of concern but also from a published study or review article in a similar area. Browsing a current journal either from a clinical specialty area or research journal such as the *Australian Journal of Advanced Nursing* or key references provided by a known expert, may provide you with a launching pad for further relevant literature.

Networking is an extremely useful technique, in that most articles reporting research contain a literature review. Do not overlook the importance of studies already used by another author. A complex, though systematic method of networking is described by O'Connor (1992). The importance of being able to recognise the link from one piece of research to another is well illustrated. The bibliography may often lead you to a much needed research tool or clinical instrument. Known experts and studies will also assist you to select appropriate review articles, as familiar authors and researchers will be recognised as being highly relevant.

Searching the literature

Once you have selected your topic, formulated your research questions, refined your search strategy with regard to the limitations and scope of your topic, and utilised all the known sources of information, the challenge that remains is to identify the unknown sources of information.

The search for the unknown relies on skills using secondary sources, such as printed indexes, the library catalogue and electronic forms such as compact disc (CD-ROM) or dial-up (on-line) technology.

You may consider performing the search yourself. This is certainly encouraged, though I would urge you to seek assistance from a professional information manager, such as your local health or university librarian. The aim would be to have this expert perhaps validate or guide your decisions related to choice of database, search strategies, combinations of terms, etc. It is most effective for you to work side by side with a librarian to ensure the optimum results are achieved. If you choose to have the search performed by an intermediary, fees may be charged.

Using the catalogue

If you have direct access to a library catalogue, either in a university, hospital or health centre, it will be well worth a search on your topic. It could be argued that the content of books may be too old. However, you may identify an excellent source of theoretical information or find a bibliography that might refer you to other key resources or alert you to key researchers in the field of study. It may be a useful avenue to identify a book on *Instruments for Clinical Nursing Research* such as the one edited by Marilyn Frank-Stromberg (1992). You may also find other resources of interest, such as conference proceedings, theses or relevant audio-visual resources.

Most library catalogues are now automated, known as OPACs (On-line Public Access Catalogues) and will facilitate searching under your broad identified key words, such as pain, sleep or surgery. Remember though, this type of search will only identify resources held in that library or, perhaps, group of libraries (many hospitals and universities are co-operating by providing joint databases). To identify all relevant literature on your topic, it is important to explore other indexes and databases.

Using journal indexes

There are a wide variety of printed indexes and abstracting services available. It is certainly sound practice to search these initially to identify some key references and gain a feel for the literature already available on the topic.

The indexes are most useful when you have perhaps a single concept to search such as 'post-operative pain', 'hallucinations' or 'sleep disorders'.

Your choice of printed indexes is varied ranging from specialised nursing indexes, including *International Nursing Index* (INI) and CINAHL, to biomedical coverage in *Index Medicus*, psychological coverage in *Psychological Abstracts* and sociological coverage in tools such as ASSIA (*Applied Social Sciences Index and Abstracts*).

Australian data can also be searched using the printed APAIS (Australian Public Affairs Information Service) index which includes journals such as the *Australian Nurses' Journal*. This listing is particularly useful for the retrieval of conference proceedings and government publications. APAIS can also be helpful for search topics more community based, such as 'remote area nursing', though it is of limited use for resources on post-operative care where the heading is likely to be 'surgery' (a very broad heading).

The Australian coverage in all mentioned international indexes is relatively good in the areas of health, nursing and medicine, although it is often difficult to find. The CINAHL does include a geographic subheading though used sparingly and rarely for clinical topics. Other helpful unique features include the use of descriptors, such as 'research' or 'case study' and the inclusion of the number of citations included in each article's bibliography, giving an indication of how substantial the article is (Shockley 1988).

A useful feature of the INI (for the years 1986-1991) is the 'Nursing Citation Index'. A citation index can be useful to work forward from a given article. This has been particularly useful to search for current articles related to nurse theorists (often initiated in literature perhaps ten or twenty years ago). Developments in electronic searching have overtaken this index, though the concept of a citation index is worthwhile to keep in mind.

Be aware that both the INI and *Index Medicus* contain foreign language articles, listed after the English language articles. The foreign items are enclosed in [square] brackets, with the language of publication following the citation. Neither of the key indexes containing clinical related research (other than in psychology or more specialised medical disciplines) have abstracts, so you are limited by the keyword access you have chosen and the title of the article (reinforcing the need for research titles and related publication titles to be meaningful).

As you will require recent clinical research articles, it is important to search the most recent monthly issues first then work back through each annual volume. You will find overlap between articles indexed in the key sources mentioned, so only search *Index Medicus* if you need additional biomedical literature. A good researcher will search both the INI and the CINAHL.

If you are familiar with searching a particular index, you will be able to transfer your skills to another index, as the features and format are essentially the same. Indexes are generally arranged alphabetically by subject with an author listing. This is particularly useful if you have been alerted to a specific researcher in the field or need to verify some incomplete bibliographic detail (such as correct dates or volume numbers). You have already been introduced to the several subject headings lists or thesauruses available. This step will have helped you determine the existence of the term 'bed rest' as well as 'sleep' or 'perioperative care' as well as 'postoperative pain'.

A search of the printed index INI could successfully and quickly help you to identify a relevant article. The example of the listing generated during a search of the term 'sleep disorders' depicted in Figure 2.1 illustrates the important features of an index entry.

Article title	*Author*
Sleep patterns and stress in patients having coronary bypass. Knapp-Spooner C, et al Heart Lung 1992 Jul-Aug; 21(4):342-9 (12 REF)	

Journal Title Abbreviation	*Date*	*Volume*	*Issue*	*Pages*	*Number of citations in reference list*

Fig. 2.1 Extract from the *International Nursing Index*

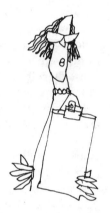

Take note that the abbreviated title may not be sufficient for you to locate the journal, e.g. *Australian Journal of Advanced Nursing* is seen as 'Aust J Adv Nurs', *Clinical Nurse Specialist* as 'Clin Nurs Spec'. If this is the case, consult the front of each volume where a list of full titles is usually to be found.

Be aware also that the bibliographic format may not be consistent with that required for your research report. In the given example, the author, Knapp-Spooner, would usually be entered before the title in your review. To be safe, write down all the information given and then later select the relevant references and rearrange them in the prescribed format.

Searching printed indexes is not particularly difficult, provided you choose appropriate keywords (using lists of subject headings to assist) and systematically work through each volume of each index. Try to keep a record of the terms you have used, the indexes you have searched, including the dates and the detail of the articles you want to pursue further.

Indexes are less effective if you need to find literature related to several concepts, covering several years and, perhaps, several disciplines. For example the sample problem identified earlier, 'The relationship between the healing process and the experiences of pain and sleep in the elderly patient undergoing surgery', would be searched far more effectively using electronic systems.

Electronic searching

An electronic literature search is a process whereby you identify in specific terms what information you need, choose the database most likely to contain it, access the database through a computer and examine the literature related to your topic' (Kilby & McAlindon 1992).

The most common bibliographic databases contain citations to journal articles, theses, books or other primary or secondary literature. Others may include references to documents such as technical reports, audio-visual materials or computer software packages. There are also a variety of electronic options, including direct online access, computer software packages or CD-ROM (Compact Disc-Read Only Memory).

Access to online databases requires: a microcomputer, a telephone line, a modem, a communications card with appropriate connecting cables and communications software. The most frequent database utilised by health workers in this way is Medline, a computerised version of *Index Medicus*, with access to the *International Nursing Index* and the *Index to Dental Literature*. CINAHL, ERIC and PsycINFO have also been utilised in this manner; access being facilitated by commercial vendors such as the Dialog Information Retrieval Service. Several useful Australian networks are also available, including Ozline which provides access to the *Australasian Medical Index* (AMI). This database, which began in 1985, provides access to indexed articles published in Australia and New Zealand.

Developed specialised software packages (often referred to as front-end or end-user) are available for do-it-yourself searching. These include GratefulMed and Paperchase (to access Medline) and Nursesearch (based on CINAHL). While these packages may be easy to use, they often do not have complete coverage nor provide intensive search capabilities and so are generally not as thorough or effective as online or CD-ROM searching.

Almost without exception, the key databases across all disciplines are now available in CD-ROM format, including Medline, CINAHL, PsycLIT, ERIC and Austrom. A range of commercial vendors produce these databases on CD-ROM, and though the content and structure of each one should be the same, the computer software and command language will differ. For example, Medline on Silver Platter will look slightly different on Dialog, Ebsco, CDPlus or Compact Cambridge, the most frequently acquired formats. The judgement of where to search remains with you, the individual researcher, and though they are designed to be user friendly, practice and perseverance is often required to successfully use the system. You should have access to a CD-ROM service in most libraries, many provide local area networks (LANs), giving many users access to many databases simultaneously.

The strength of searching electronically is often seen as compensation for the inadequacies of searching printed indexes. You will, for instance:

- have greater flexibility in relation to free text searching
- be able to limit your search in a variety of ways, often over several years at one time (a great time saver which may result in an accurate, relevant, exhaustive search within minutes)
- be able to obtain abstracts for many of the citations (hence, better able to judge the article as the abstract will give a far greater indication of validity and context than is possible with the title only)
- be able to search a number of different concepts simultaneously (i.e. the ability to link and combine terms).

There is also the opportunity for 'serendipitous discovery of data related to your topic' (Kilby & McAlindon 1992).

What will a search result look like? The sample result from a search of a bibliographic database for literature on the topic related to pain and sleep following surgery (as shown in Fig. 2.2) resembles a citation from the printed index, with the added feature of an abstract.

Most database entries resemble this record, with description tags for each field abbreviated. (In this example, TI stands for title, AU for author, AD for address of author, SO for source; the journal title—vital information to retrieve the complete article, ISSN for International Standard Serial Number, PY for publication year, LA for language, CP for country of publication, AB for abstract.)

Successful steps to electronic searching. There are several useful steps to assist you in effectively searching a database.

Plan your search. Remember to state your topic clearly, decide where to search, what type of documents are needed, etc. A worksheet or search planner sheet is recommended to help you describe and plan your search, listing terms and their relationships to each other.

Translate your topic into searchable terms. As with printed index searching, a thesaurus can be of great assistance. The advantage of a database is that you may have access to an automated thesaurus, searchable from an index or similar file.

Connect the terms you have listed. This requires an understanding of 'logical operators' or 'Boolean connectors', the most common being AND, OR and NOT. Consider our sample search: The connector OR is used to join the similar terms 'sleep' OR 'insomnia' and will retrieve items that discuss either concept, as shown in Figure 2.3. This process *broadens* your search.

The connector AND is used to link different concepts, such as 'sleep' AND 'pain' and will only retrieve articles about both terms, as shown in Figure 2.4. This process *refines* your search.

TI: Patients' night-time pain, analgesic provision and sleep after surgery.
AU: Closs-SJ
AD: Department of Nursing Studies, University of Edinburgh, U.K.
SO: Int-J-Nurs-Stud. 1992 Nov; 29(4): 381-92
ISSN: 0020-7489
PY: 1992
LA: ENGLISH
CP: ENGLAND
AB: One hundred patients were interviewed about their experiences of pain and sleep following abdominal surgery. This information was supplemented by data on analgesic provision which were gathered from medication charts. Pain was the most commonly reported cause of night-time sleep disturbance and analgesics helped more patients to get back to sleep than any other intervention. About half of the patients felt that pain was worse at night than during the day...

Fig. 2.2 Extract from a bibliographic database

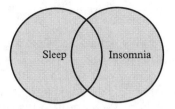
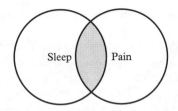

Fig. 2.3 Result of using 'OR' to connect terms. Shading indicates area searched.

Fig. 2.4 Result of using 'AND' to connect terms. Shading indicates area searched.

It is essential you write each step (on your planner) in the order you will enter them into the computer. Keep the search statements simple and avoid confusing the connectors in one statement. For example, the search statements could resemble:

Statement 1: sleep OR bed rest OR insomnia
Statement 2: surgery OR postoperative care OR preoperative care
Statement 3: 1 AND 2 AND pain

As a general rule, avoid using different connectors in the same statement. If you choose to do so however, adhere to the order of precedence by using AND before OR, if in the same statement.

Implement strategies to refine or limit your search. This will require the use of the AND operator. If you only need articles about 'pain' in a given year, enter pain AND py=1993. Some useful limit factors include:

- limit to particular dates (can often use for a single year, as shown above, or a range of years, e.g. py>1990)
- limit to English publications only
- limit to research documents or publications of a particular type, e.g. pain AND research in dt (where dt = document type, pt used for publication type).

Implement other strategies to ensure an efficient search statement. Most systems allow you to truncate terms (often using the symbol ⋆) or to use a 'wild card' (such as ?) particularly if variant spelling is possible. For example if you want:

- articles on Australia, Australian, use Austral⋆
- to cater for US spelling, use p?ediatrics, orthop?edics, organi?ation, etc.

Do be cautious though, as some shortcuts may retrieve unwanted terms, e.g. nurs⋆ will retrieve nurseries, nursing homes, nurses, or (depending on the database) even totally unrelated concepts such as nursery-rhymes.

Know the system you are using (each will vary slightly) to enable you to:
- display a full record
- sort records, either by journal title or author

- print records (often you need to tell the system precisely which fields you need)
- download the records, (rather than printing) if you have access to a computer to then organise and annotate your records.

Remember at this point, it might be useful to save your search strategy in case you decide to search another database. Alternatively, you may be ready to move on and locate and assess the quality of the complete research article.

Selecting, locating and organising the articles

Once you have successfully identified a list of articles relevant to your topic, it is time to select the most relevant to read more fully and perhaps use in your literature review. If you have refined and limited your search adequately, you will have a manageable list. More than one hundred items is becoming excessive, though need will differ depending on focus of search. The emphasis should be on quality, not quantity.

Selection of relevant articles

At this point, you need to recall the aim of the literature review. You may read more articles than you actually need to include in the final proposal or research report. The selected articles should be relevant to the research problem, contain mostly primary sources and provide a rationale for the research.

Some useful guidelines described by Sackett (1981) include

- the title, is it interesting, does it look useful?
- the authors, do they have a good track record, are they familiar?
- the summary (or abstract), is it informative, does it relate to your own study (in terms of the subject, the setting and the sample). Is it interesting?

Be careful to exclude any foreign articles (unless you are prepared to use only the abstract or obtain a translation). Also, you may consider giving some preference to refereed journals which are highly reputable in their specialty area. These are often indicated in the abstract or on the journal itself.

Organising your records

You need to keep a record (perhaps on small cards) of relevant articles identified in your initial search. Most likely, you will have a print-out of the articles retrieved from the CD-ROM search, sorted alphabetically by title of journal (to speed up the process of locating the articles). The ideal is to transfer the sorted data from the CD-ROM search, to a disk for transfer to a compatible word processing package or database such as Procite (design-ed to organise and manage bibliographic information). To this database, you could add other data identified from non-electronic searching. It is recommended you re-sort the records alphabetically by author, awaiting arrival of the article or compilation of photocopies and in preparation for the final review step. Either way, you need to be able to annotate each entry as you retrieve it, scan it and make judgements as to its value. The systematic recording of references can be demanding, though will save valuable time and effort (especially if you misplace information and need to repeat searching).

Choosing collections and services

Once you have completed your search you will need to learn how to find your way past the library's reference collection where the dictionaries, directories and printed indexes and the CD-ROM service are usually housed. You also need to know what other forms of delivery are available if the library does not hold the item you need.

There are many sophisticated library services, probably right on your doorstep. It will pay to find out what access you can gain, particularly to university and major hospital and health libraries *before* you attempt to obtain your articles. You will be able to judge suitability of the article far more efficiently if you are able to scan the journal before photocopying. Very rarely, though, will any one library carry all the primary resources you need to obtain. Be reassured, however, that libraries are in the business of providing pathways to the literature in the quickest, most cost effective manner. This may include system network access, joint catalogues or the provision of union lists such as that provided by the GRATIS network of libraries in South Australia, Queensland and Victoria or the Joint Serials list for health libraries in Western Australia.

It will help too if you know how the library collec-tion is arranged. Most will use a standard classi-fication system such as the Dewey Decimal System (DDC) where surgical information, for example, will be found mostly at 617, or the National Library of Medicine Scheme (NLM), involving an A–Z type classification, where surgical information, for instance, will be found at WO100. Classification systems are, essentially, employed to help you by grouping 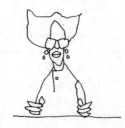 resources on a similar topic together. Journals or serials literature will be classified in a similar manner in larger libraries, usually in a separate section from books or audio-visual (AV) or microform (MF) or reference items (usually identified by an R). In smaller libraries, it is usual to shelve journals alphabetically, by title.

Ask the library staff to describe the inter-library loan service available to you. It is a vital pathway to assist you in obtaining articles out of town.

Electronic delivery

Most libraries now use electronic network systems to locate and retrieve particular items not purchased by that library. The Australian Bibliographic Network (ABN) is a national database used throughout Australia to identify which libraries hold a particular item. Electronic mail systems are then frequently used to request the item to be copied, sent by facsimile or borrowed.

The world wide Internet system (a computer based network) is now making it possible for you to locate an item on an overseas database, request it electronically and have the item faxed to you, often within a working day. Most universities and some hospitals in Australia are members of the Australian Academic and Research Network (AARNet) which, through a satellite link from Melbourne to California, is part of the Internet. Increasingly, more journals will be accessible electronically.

Many libraries are also providing actual complete journals in electronic format, often called a full text document storage system, usually on CD-ROM. The National Library of Australia has a system called ADONIS (which includes journals such as *Lancet, British Medical Journal* and *Pain*). The CD-ROM database, known as HealthROM, an initiative of the Australian Department of Health, Housing, Local Government and Community Services, is being developed to cover the areas of public and environmental health, drug and alcohol abuse, HIV/AIDS and other communicable diseases. In addition to providing databases of journal citations, including the *Australasian Medical Index* (AMI), it contains many full text publications, mostly government documents, such as papers related to the National Health Strategy or papers published by the National Health and Medical Research Council.

Costs involved

Many services are now demanding a fee, so be prepared to budget for costs such as photocopying, electronic searching and electronic delivery. Even if you conduct the search yourself, fees may be charged if you need to obtain the article from overseas. Many services, such as those accessible via AARNet, now make provision for use of Mastercard or Visa card payment. Copying from full text services may also cost more than standard photocopies from printed journals, as copyright and royalty payments are required.

Writing the literature review

Your aim is to now present the literature review logically and conclude with a summary, appraising the quality of the literature, identifying knowledge gaps and giving an indication of directions for future research. The final review can be organised in a variety of ways, usually by concepts related to the problem investigated.

The process of systematically searching, selecting and organising the literature as described in this chapter will go a long way toward maintaining the aim of the literature review and securing a sound focus for the further development of your own research project.

REFERENCES

Burns N 1987 The practice of nursing research: conduct, critique and utilisation. Saunders, Philadelphia
Frank-Stromberg M (ed) 1992 Instruments for clinical nursing research. Jones & Bartlett, Boston
Kilby S A, McAlindon M N 1992 Searching the literature yourself: why how and what to search. In: Arnold J M (ed) Computer application in nursing education, pub. no. 14–2406. National League for Nursing, New York
O'Connor S E 1992 Network theory: a systematic method for literature review. Nurse Education Today 12:44–50
Sackett D L 1981 How to read clinical journals. Canadian Medical Association Journal 124:555–558
Shockley J S (ed) 1988 Information sources for nursing, a guide, pub. no. 41–2200. National League for Nursing, New York

3. Winning finance for your project

Helen Hamilton

Applying for a grant is a bit like entering a competition. There are conditions to be met to be eligible for entry, and criteria for judging entries. Only a few entrants will be winners, but the rules are the same for everyone, whether novice or expert. As in most competitions, the judges' decision is final. The difference between winning financial assistance for research and a lottery is that it is skill, rather than luck, which increases the chance of success. Those applying for funds should understand that it is a highly competitive business and in it, the written application has a critical role. For this reason it is essential for you to be able to present your ideas well in writing—because it is on what is written that the judges make decisions. This chapter is directed towards those who are new to the task of developing and writing proposals and those who have learnt that they need to develop their skills in this area. The aim is to provide insight into the nature of grant proposals and to offer suggestions which will enhance your skills in grant proposal writing.

Expectations of funding bodies

As the sponsors of nursing research projects, funding agencies have the responsibility to ensure that funds are allocated to studies which not only have the potential to be successfully completed, but also are likely to make a significant contribution. Therefore, when 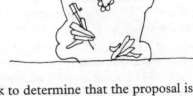 assessing applications, reviewers will seek to determine that the proposal is not only achievable, but also consistent with the goals of the funding body. The factors on which such decisions are based are discussed below.

Relevance to funding agency

The relevance of the proposed application to the aims of the funding agency is usually the first criterion to be assessed. Reviewers will therefore expect the proposal to show how the aims of the proposed research are congruent with those of the funding agency. If an application is not within the interests of an agency it will proceed no further in the review process.

Significance of the research

Another important criterion relates to the value of the research itself. During the review process the question will be asked, 'Is this study worth doing?' To a large extent the answer will depend on how well you can convey the importance of your proposal. As a matter of course, reviewers will expect to see a convincing description of either the expected impact, the study outcome, or what will change as a result. What you write about the significance of the research and its benefits is highly relevant to the assessment of the worth of the study. In particular, reviewers appreciate the researcher's ability to foresee outcomes and the skill with which this is conveyed in the application.

Ability of researcher

During the review process an assessment will also be made of your capacity to carry out the proposed study. While past experience and qualifications are important, they are not the only indicators of competence. Your grasp of the topic; understanding of likely problems and how these will be overcome, avoided or nullified; and the overall quality of the application itself are all assessed when reviewers judge a researcher's ability to successfully carry out the study they propose.

Appropriateness of the method

Reviewers will expect you to show in a detailed description of the research design that you have complete mastery over your proposed method. They will also judge your competence as a researcher by evaluating the appropriateness of your chosen method to the nature of the study. In other words 'Is the study, as planned, the most appropriate way to answer the question asked?' There are many ways to conduct research inquiries. Not all phenomena are amenable to being reduced to numbers and statistics and some will be more appropriately approached using qualitative methods. The test is: 'Will the method selected generate data which can be relied upon to inform about the topic?' In this regard the match between the topic being explored and the method proposed to collect data is critical.

As researchers are expected to be rigorous in their work, reviewers will also seek out evidence in your proposal as to how you will act to avoid or correct any identified weaknesses in the study—to ensure that the end result can be relied on.

Feasibility of the study

A range of practical considerations to do with the successful implementation and conduct of the study also form part of the evaluation process. These include an assessment of whether:

- the time allowed for the study is realistic and in keeping with its size and complexity;
- the population of people/things to be included in the study is accessible in the time frame specified;
- any necessary pre-study activities have been identified and included in the research plan.

As these aspects are critical to the successful conduct of any research project, it will be expected that these and other practical issues will be addressed in the proposal in sufficient detail so as to confirm the feasibility of the study.

Appropriate assessment of resources

Reviewers will not simply assume that you have been accurate, careful and cognisant of the need to minimise the demand for human and material resources during the development of your proposal. Consequently they will be looking for evidence in your application which adequately justifies the resources you are asking for.

Ethical considerations

As meticulous compliance with ethical standards is mandatory, reviewers will expect to see how the ethical aspects of the study are to be dealt with. Funding agencies normally require documented evidence that the proposed study has been approved by the appropriate Institutional Ethics Committee/s. Some may even expect purpose designed forms to be completed and attached to the application.

Presentation

While the content of the proposal is of the utmost importance, the presentation of an application can also influence its chance of success—particularly if it is found to be incomplete or illegible. In this regard, reviewers will expect that all the required documentation has been provided, and that details of the study are legibly presented in a logical sequence.

Compiling a grant application

With a knowledge of the expectations of funding agencies, you will be in a better position to begin putting together your proposal. Even with this knowledge however, writing a grant application is not something which can be achieved quickly. It takes considerable time and energy to address each of the issues described below and compile a competitive proposal. Failure to do so will usually have an adverse influence on the quality of your proposal and its prospects for success.

Clarifying your thoughts

Research ideas have to mature. This means that an intellectual process of evolution must take place in the researcher's mind until a point is reached where the nature of the problem is fully understood, and a clear focus and direction for a study becomes evident. For most people this process cannot be hurried. A proposal written prematurely will be an unsatisfactory one, because it will fail to provide the conceptual depth that reviewers seek 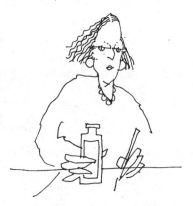 as a demonstration of the applicant's intellectual grasp of the undertaking.

Actually it is necessary to be fairly well advanced in thinking about the project, and how it might be carried out, *before* you put pen to paper. What is sometimes called the 'conceptual phase' of development is fully completed before proposal writing begins. In practice this means that all the processes of reading, thinking, writing and talking about the topic are pursued until a clear understanding of what is to be studied and why, and the most appropriate way to carry it out, emerges. Beginning researchers have difficulty in judging their level of preparedness for writing and here an experienced mentor can provide invaluable assistance. As a rough guide, however, you will know that you have reached an advanced stage when you can unhesitatingly state the purpose of the inquiry or the research question(s), why it should be answered, and what approach you will take to carry out the study and why. When this is clear there is yet another set of issues—associated with implementing the project—which must be considered before you can begin writing the proposal.

Confirming the feasibility of the study

As soon as the intellectual process has given form and substance to the project, its feasibility should be explored on a much more practical level.

There are several things to consider in assessing whether a project is feasible or not. No matter how skilfully conceptualised a project is, it may nevertheless founder if the practical aspects of the study are not considered early in the development of the project. As a matter of course reviewers will look for evidence in your application which demonstrates that attention has been given to the aspects discussed below.

Ethical considerations

The proposed study must comply with the ethical principles which protect individuals from harm and preserve dignity in research situations. Careful consideration of any ethical concerns the study raises should occur prior to writing the proposal which should ultimately include a description of how participants will be:

- recruited to the study;
- presented with information which will ensure consent to participate is informed;
- informed of their rights as participants in the research—including the right to withdraw from the study;
- advised of the research findings.

Studies must be deemed ethically sound *before* the proposal is submitted to the funding agency. All major tertiary hospitals and universities have IECs set up for the purpose of ensuring research proposals comply with ethical standards. Ethical clearance is essential for all research proposals and, if the research is carried out in more than one setting, from each IEC. A planning hint is to know when Institutional Ethics Committees (IECs) meetings are scheduled in your proposed research setting/s so that you can include this step in your time plan. (See Ch. 4.)

Co-operation of other groups

Many studies require the assistance of other individuals or groups to carry them out. For example, suppose a new nursing technique is to be evaluated against the standard procedure to see if it provides a better outcome. This study design requires random assignment of subjects to treatment or control groups, and its success will depend on nurses in the research setting following procedures prescribed by the research protocol. In these circumstances the co-operation of the staff in implementing the research requirements is essential. Negotiating the necessary assistance may take time and, in some situations, may even necessitate the implementation of educational programs for those collaborating in the research. When appropriate, an indication that this aspect of the study has been considered should be included in the proposal.

Access to participants for the study

Where nursing research is to be undertaken in clinical or other institutions, it is essential that you negotiate permission to conduct the study with the appropriate people in the selected research setting *prior* to writing your proposal. You may even find that some funding agencies require a part of the application form be completed and signed by a responsible person in the proposed location. Alternatively, letters from key individuals, which acknowledge that support for your study has been successfully negotiated, may be included.

In addition to permission to use the location, there are other aspects of access to consider. For example, it is relatively easy at the conceptual stage, to describe the people who will take part in the study. What is sometimes more difficult is locating and contacting them. For example, if a study is to include 75 year old male patients, with non insulin dependent diabetes, who developed deep vein thromboses post elective inguinal hernia repairs, how would you find them? Using diagnosis as the identifier, it is relatively easy where computerised inpatient lists are available. But who controls access to the computerised lists? And how can they be found if no lists are available? Issues of this type must be explored and settled *before* submitting the application, which should indicate how the study population will be accessed.

A related question is, 'Can the *number* of people specified be accessed?' If, for example, 500 respondents are to be included, then you must be confident that that number can be found in the time frame for the study. Working out whether or not the number of people who meet the criteria for the study can be found may involve some preliminary investigative work on your part (see Ch. 5). It is time well spent however—to avoid the embarrassment of failing to complete a study, or completing it inadequately due to an absence of participants. (Neither of these would look well in a final report to the funding agency.) It is essential for you to know that respondents are available and accessible and to reflect this information in your proposal.

Assessment of resources

It is important to have a detailed and complete understanding of the resources, physical, financial and human, that your study will require. If, for example, you wish to evaluate a new, recently marketed dressing for leg ulcers, it will be necessary to know, not only the cost of the dressings, but also that the supply is assured. A study of this type may include only 'clean' ulcers and therefore swabs will need to be taken for culture to ensure that infected ulcers are excluded. Not only the time and equipment for taking the swabs will be costed, but also the laboratory processing of the swabs taken for culture. Funding agencies require applicants to justify the items in the budget. This means they want you to explain the costs claimed and to show why they are necessary. It is worth remembering that budgets are always very closely scrutinised, particularly personnel and equipment items, as these tend to be the costliest outlays.

If the research proposed depends upon using an expensive piece of equipment, or requires expensive procedures, then you may have to think again if you are a beginner. Funding agencies are unlikely to support costly budgets from applicants with no proven research record, no matter how well justified. In these instances, you should look for alternative ways of approaching the problem.

It is good practice to identify *all* cost items before proceeding with cost estimates. Do not forget to include any consultants' fees (e.g. laboratory technicians, statisticians) if you need their assistance. More information on costing is provided in the discussion on budget in the section on writing the proposal.

Choosing a funding agency

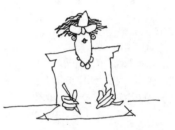

With a good understanding of what you propose to study and how it will be carried out, you can consider approaching a funding agency. The first step to success in funding is to be certain that the research proposed lies within the interests of the agency where you wish to apply. Most researchers seek the common ground between their own research interests and those of an agency and shape the proposal accordingly. As the choice of an agency strongly influences the selection of topic, the selection of an appropriate funding body should be an early consideration in the development of any project for which financial assistance is required.

Part of the knowledge base for researchers is a good understanding of who has money available for research and for what purposes. Knowledge of this sort is usually 'picked up' rather than taught. Most universities have research offices which collect this kind of information and make it available to staff and students. Others may find publications such as directories or other listings helpful in locating agencies. What you need to know to choose a appropriate agency is identified next.

Purpose of the funding

Every funding agency has particular purposes for which it makes money available. Part of the art of making successful grant applications is to select an agency with research interests that match the aims of your proposed study. To make the point, it is no use applying to an agency whose research interests are patients with cancer if the planned study is concerned with a population of patients with asthma. This example is exaggerated of course;

in reality the distinctions are not usually so obvious. It is quite acceptable to discuss your research with an agency before making an application, to ascertain the interest of the agency in the proposed work. It is also helpful to know what studies the agency has funded previously.

It is probably appropriate to note at this point, that although there are many ways to carry out research, the techniques which use numbers and statistics (i.e. quantitative ones) are those which have the widest acceptance among funding agencies. If you are planning a study which is not going to use the numbers approach (i.e. qualitative research), it would be prudent to ask the funding agency whether they will accept it *before* submitting an application.

Value of research awards

As the value of research awards varies from a hundred dollars or less—to tens of thousands of dollars, it is important to know the value of awards so that appropriate requests can be made. Clearly if a proposed study requires $10 000, you will need to be confident that the selected agency makes awards of this value. If commencement is dependent on the provision of funding, it will also be necessary to know when successful applicants can expect to be paid, and whether the money will be paid all at once, or in instalments. The latter can have implications for planning the conduct of the study.

Eligibility and availability

Most funding agencies specify who is eligible to apply for awards. Some are discipline specific, that is the applicant must be, for example, a medical practitioner, or a registered nurse, to be eligible to receive an award. In addition, conditions may be imposed on the availability of funds. For example, it is often the case that money provided by private donors is conditional on the sum being allowed as a tax deductible donation. In these cases it will be necessary to know whether grants of money for research purposes made to your selected organisation can be claimed as a tax deduction by the donor.

Prior to submitting your application, you must be confident that you can meet any specific requirements set by the funding agency. Proof of eligibility will usually be required before any award is finalised.

Conditions for grants

It is usual for funding agencies to require researchers to agree to standard conditions if they are successful in their application. Such provisions may cover matters such as reporting procedures on the part of the researcher to the agency during the conduct of the study; ownership of any equipment paid for by the award; conditions under which funds will be terminated; and financial accounting procedures and other relevant matters. Standard conditions are usually supplied with application forms, however many agencies will reserve the right to impose other conditions if there is a particular concern about a proposal.

By signing the application form, researchers agree to abide by the conditions of the grant. Should you accept a grant you will be expected to know the conditions under which it is made—as you will be accountable for adhering to the terms and conditions.

Application procedures and processing

Once you have decided where to apply for funding, you should obtain an application form. Knowing the requirements of your chosen agency will help you order your thinking about the project and assist you to develop a fully rounded proposal. While government sources always have application forms which are detailed in the direction they provide, other agencies may only provide guidelines. In these cases following the model provided by government forms is a good idea, to make sure nothing is omitted from the application.

It is also in your interest to learn as much as possible from the agency about the processing of applications, the closing date for submissions and the name and address of the person to whom you are to send your application. Most funding agencies have standard procedures for processing grants, and this can be useful information. An awareness of the stages of the review process, and who the reviewers are likely to be can provide you with an understanding of your audience and allow you to shape your application accordingly.

Writing grant proposals

Structuring a grant proposal is greatly assisted when application forms are available. They assist researchers to provide all the information that a funding agency needs to assess the proposal. Even with this guidance however, just what to write can still be a dilemma. Broadly speaking, the information required in grant proposals falls into two categories—details about the researcher/s and a comprehensive plan of the proposed research.

Researcher's profile

The sort of information you will be required to supply about yourself will include basic details such as your name, address, contact telephone/facsimile numbers and current occupation. Your curriculum vitae should reflect your research background and include reference to:

(a) research experience—list the titles of studies you have been part of and the role you had in carrying them out such as research assistant; senior researcher; principal researcher;

(b) education—list your research qualifications and your formal research education. Add any additional courses in methodology or postgraduate diplomas involving research, research units completed in courses; degrees by research;

(c) publications—provide a list of studies you have published in the past and/or whether earlier studies have been implemented or findings used in any way;

(d) previous support—mention any funding you have received for previous research studies and name the source/s. No matter the size of the grant, it is the fact that others have had confidence in your work to give you money, that is the point.

Description of the proposed study

The information researchers supply about themselves and the manner of writing and presentation forms the basis of judging the competence of the researcher—and their ability to carry out what is proposed. While this information is essential to the review process, the component of the application which carries the most weight is the information supplied about the proposed study. Although the details required may vary from agency to agency, some categories of information are common to all grant proposals. These are discussed in the following pages.

Project title. The title is an indication to the reader of what the study is about. It therefore must be both specific and descriptive of the proposed study. It is not appropriate to use abbreviated titles or to depart from the traditional format of descriptive style when applying for grants. In this situation the title is expected to do the job of reflecting what the study is about, so that the reader is oriented to what is to come.

Background to the study. The sections discussed under this general heading should allow for the logical development of the study from the context of its beginning to the justification for the direction of its focus. 'Background' is understood to include the following information:

Introduction. Picking up the lead given in the title, the opening remarks will expand on the subject of the study. Explained will be how the subject came to be noticed. This might be the result of a preliminary investigation of the topic; earlier research; observation and reading and experience in the field, or all of these. The introduction is brief but sufficient to provide a context for the purpose of the research.

Purpose of the research. The purpose of the proposed study can be expressed as a statement or a question. Either way it is crucial to provide an unequivocal indication of what the study is about. A sentence beginning 'The purpose of this study is ...' or 'The question for this study is ...' *must* be included. Although this seems obvious, a surprising number of researchers neglect to provide the focus for their study in this way. Its importance can be understood when it is realised that other critical judgements of the proposal, such as the appropriateness of the method, depend upon this information. To fail to express the purpose of the study adequately will leave the proposal without a focus and liable to being dismissed by reviewers as 'weak', 'underdeveloped', 'unclear' or 'vague.'

Rationale. Reasons are given in support of the purpose for the study as to why the research should be carried out. This is called 'the rationale for the study'. It is sometimes separate to the purpose of the study, but in the examples given below the purpose and rationale are expressed together.

1. The concept of the hospice in [Australia] has evolved in the last decade. The research literature related to this kind of care is sparse. No one has systematically determined what hospice care givers actually do. Furthermore, no research has been conducted to ascertain from terminally ill persons and their families what it is that hospice care givers do that constitutes effective care. Therefore, the [purpose] of this descriptive study is *to identify the effective and ineffective behaviours of hospice care givers in providing care to terminally ill persons and their families in a home setting.*
2. Knowledge of one's state of health is a pre-requisite for practising self-care. A lack of knowledge has consequences that may seriously affect biological integrity and quality of cancer patients' lives when they are receiving radiation therapy. To date, no comprehensive anticipatory approach has been tried to help patients prevent or manage the side effects of radiation therapy before their development. The [purpose] for the proposed experimental study is *to test the effectiveness of presenting side effect management techniques information before the occurrence of experienced side effects on care behaviours.*
3. The [purpose] for this study is to expand the body of knowledge about the experience of pain in adolescents. The long-range goal is to provide health professionals with information to enable them to deal more effectively with adolescents who are anticipating or experiencing pain. The specific study question is, '*Do adolescents hospitalized for acute or chronic illness describe the pain experience the same as non hospitalised adolescents?*'

(Adapted from Wilson H 1985 p 197)

In each example a reasoned justification is given in support of the purpose of the study. The indication for the focus of the study is given clearly and distinguished further by the use of italics. This use of visual devices draws the readers' attention to the key points, thus leaving them in no doubt about what is to be studied.

Objectives for the study. The objectives should be logically related to the purpose for the study. In stating these, you are indicating what the study will achieve. Objectives may take the form of a set of related questions to be answered in the study or, when appropriate, related hypotheses to be tested.

Literature review. There are several purposes for the literature review. Reviewing literature relevant to the topic for the proposed research expands the explanation and justification for the purpose and/or design of a study. Where appropriate it can provide the theoretical basis for the hypotheses to be tested and definitions of key concepts. Literature reviews, done well, present the reader with an overview of the current knowledge of the topic and critical evaluation, that is the strengths and limitations of the studies included. Comparing what is proposed with what has been done previously will place your study in the context of current knowledge and demonstrate where it will make a contribution to improving or expanding what is known. Where limitations in previous studies are noted, you should indicate how these will be avoided or overcome in the proposed study. As a general rule, use the literature selectively to develop the theoretical and logical basis for your study. Writing all that is known about the topic is not required.

Significance of the project. Funding agencies like to know that the support they provide for researchers has worthwhile results. For this reason they ask applicants to state how important the research they propose is in terms of what benefits will ensue as a result of the investigation. It is up to you to state what benefits may arise from your research and it is in your interest to state these as clearly and directly as possible. To achieve this end, ask yourself 'What will change as a result of my study?' The answer will help to keep the focus of your research in mind and provide reviewers with enough information to decide whether or not they agree with your claims.

The contents of the previous sections serve to inform the reviewer about what is to be studied and why. Information as to how the research is to be conducted must also be supplied.

Research plan. The purpose of this section is both to explain the plan for conducting the study and to stipulate the time frame for carrying it out. Your description will allow you to demonstrate your understanding of the method you have chosen to investigate the problem. Consequently, rather than simply saying 'An experimental design will be used', you should describe the design in detail:

An experimental design will be used; sixty people who meet the selection criteria (which have been listed and explained earlier) will be randomly assigned, thirty to a treatment and thirty to a control group. The treatment group will receive X intervention (explain the intervention fully), and the control group a placebo (explain the placebo intervention). Scores on the selected measures (name the measures and the statistical tests to be applied) will then be compared to test the null hypothesis (state the null hypothesis).

The study expressed in these terms has the advantage of providing reviewers with a good description of what is planned and gives them to understand that you know what you are about.

The following headings may be helpful as a guide as to what other aspects of the design should be included in your description of the research plan.

Preparing to collect data. Describe all preliminary activities. Include as appropriate:

- operational definitions of variables and key terms;
- development and evaluation of instruments for data collection including pilot testing;
- sampling or selection procedures including criteria for entry for participants;

- pre-testing equipment and training operators;
- development of protocols;
- a plan for any preliminary interventions or data collection required.

Collecting data. Under this heading the steps involved in the data collection process should be itemised, described and explained if necessary. This section will include as appropriate:

- a description of the research design and all aspects of bias and contamination control; or
- a description of the implementation of an alternative method of data collection.

Where the researcher is using approaches and techniques which depart from the traditional scientific methods, Hamilton and Gray (1992 p 13) recommend that as they are less well understood, full explanations of method, including theoretical assumptions, should be included.

Analysing data. Here you should describe how the data will be treated once collected. As appropriate include:

- statistical models, analyses and estimates of probability;
- details of alternative methods of data analysis/processing.

In your description of the procedures, link the plan for data analysis to the questions asked by the study.

Presenting and reporting data. Include the process of writing and producing the final report of the study and specify a date for presenting it. Plan to provide preliminary reports to the funding agency. Usually these are made when data collection begins and/or when it ends, depending on the length of the project. At least one preliminary report, if not more, are usually expected by the funding agency each year. You should therefore find out what the requirements of the agency are in this regard, and be prepared to comply with them meticulously.

If the study is large and complex, the time frame may be developed separately. Giving information about the time allowed for the study is important because reviewers like to check that enough has been allowed for each stage of the project. It serves as a guide as to how well you understand what is involved in carrying out the study.

Budget

Costing a project is usually straight forward. Successful budgeting depends on identifying and accurately estimating all human, physical and material cost factors associated with the conduct of the research. You will therefore need to obtain current quotes for equipment or other items, and use current award rates for salaries. Include in salaries/wages costs for consultants or for hiring specialised skills, e.g. statisticians; data entry/processing. Hamilton and Gray (1992 p 17) itemise the categories of resources to be considered for estimating budgets as:

Equipment
Computing
Communications
Travel
Stationery and printing
Postage
Salaries/wages (including 'on costs')
Other items peculiar to the study

These writers also warn that funding agencies are unlikely to reimburse costs which researchers can reasonably be expected to provide for themselves, e.g. things such as heating, lighting, office space. As budgets are closely scrutinised, be accurate in your estimates and reasonable in your expectations.

How to write

The qualities valued most in writing for grants come down to four: being informative; being clear; being persuasive; and doing it all in as few words as possible, that is, being succinct. What follows are suggestions as to how these qualities might be achieved.

Being informative

The objective to be achieved when writing a grant proposal is to supply reviewers with enough information for them to develop a good understanding of what is proposed and why and how it will be done. But how much is enough? Although the grant writer has to make a judgement about this, there are two extremes to avoid. One is to explain everything in so much detail that clarity is lost in an over abundance of words. The second is to assume that the reader has the same understanding as yourself and provide too little information, that is, leaving too much to be taken as understood. This is usually a costly mistake as reviewers will not attempt to read your mind—they will simply pick up the next study.

Many people find it helpful when writing to have in mind the person to whom they are writing—as a means of judging what is shared between the author and the reader. You can make use of this tactic by assuming the reader is intelligent, and knowledgeable about research procedures, but has little understanding of the specific topic you have in mind. For example, you can assume that the reviewer will know what is meant by research concepts such as 'random sample' or 'operationalisation' and so on. Knowledge of any nursing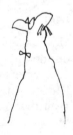

concepts in the study, however, would not be assumed. Nursing concepts such as 'nursing process' and 'nursing health assessment', for example, need to be fully explained. This is not meant to imply that reviewers will not be knowledgeable about the topic, they may be. But by imagining that they are not, you will offer a fuller and more complete explanation—this is the aim.

Conveying information effectively to a reader is a matter of both logic and language. It has as much to do with how the material is organised on the page as it does with the choice of words and content. As the order in which the writer presents the content can influence their readers' comprehension considerably, each phase of the research should be described in a logical and chronological order. The reviewer must understand, from the information provided, what the researcher intends to do, why it is to be done and how it is to be carried out. It should be a complete picture.

Being clear

A guiding principle to achieve clarity in grant writing is to keep it simple. Listed below are some suggestions as to how this can be achieved.

- *Use familiar words.* Where a familiar word will suffice use it rather than a more obscure one. Only use words or technical terms the meaning of which you are absolutely certain.
- *Be direct.* List key points as statements or use dot points for emphasis.
- *Use short sentences.* As a general rule break down long complex sentences to shorter, simpler ones to make comprehension easier for the reader.
- *Assist the reader to grasp obscure concepts.* Sometimes it is necessary to use concepts that are unfamiliar or difficult to grasp on a first reading. Do provide explanations and/or concrete examples which illustrate the idea and help to fix it in the reader's mind. Similarly, if substitutes in plain English are not feasible for technical terms use the term but include an explanation as well.
- *Avoid acronyms.* If it is necessary to use an abbreviation of this type, spell it out the first time it appears, with the acronym in brackets, as shown in the following sentence: 'In this study one hundred patients who have experienced an anterior myocardial infarction (AMI) will be interviewed.' Thereafter use the acronym in the text.
- *Use plain English rather than jargon.* Writers aim to put as few barriers between the reader and their ideas as possible. This means making yourself understood using everyday vocabulary whenever possible. Avoid pretentious language which does nothing more than inhibit understanding. These two sentences make the point:

Psychological acquiescence to subcultural values can be considered cultural contamination or attitudinal restructuring.

It should (sic) be considered that persons adapt behaviour and attitudes to the cultural values around them. (Sultz & Scherwin 1981 p 54).

These sentences say the same thing but the first is barely intelligible, and needs at least three readings to understand it. The same essential message is stated in the second, but with fewer words and less complexity. It can be understood on first reading. These are all the good qualities to achieve in writing, while the former illustrates what to avoid.

Jargon is sometimes used to imply sophistication on the part of the writer. This however often creates quite the reverse response as experienced reviewers are not impressed—just irritated.

- *Be consistent with key words.* It is important to use key words consistently in the proposal. For example, if you begin using the term 'client', keep with it throughout and avoid suddenly talking about 'patients', 'customers' or 'consumers'. Changes in key terminology distract concentration from the main narrative, by causing the reader to pause to absorb the new word and work out where it fits. Your task is to create a smooth narrative flow in the text. To reinforce the point consider 'attitudinal restructuring' suddenly appearing in the text where 'changing attitudes' was the term used earlier. A reader meeting these words half way through a proposal would be looking for the bit that was missing to explain them.
- *Be consistent in punctuation and referencing style.* It is advisable to use an acknowledged style of referencing. If you are uncertain consult a librarian. A style guide provides valuable assistance to check the finer points of punctuation. This, with a dictionary, are essential tools for all writers. Do check the spelling of all unfamiliar words and any familiar ones that are usually spelt incorrectly. Correct punctuation is essential. It facilitates meaning when it is done well. But done poorly the reviewer, at best, has to work harder to understand, and at worst, may misunderstand.
- *Attend to visual presentation.* Use strategies such as bolding, italics, small capitals and other visual devices that help organise material and draw emphasis to key points, but use them with restraint, and be consistent in their application.

Being persuasive

The best way to persuade is to build a case of sound argument that is based on fact, tempered by logic and compelling as to why your research should be carried out. It is essential to present your proposal as a reasoned piece of written work. To be convincing, it must be consistent in its internal logic. Persuasiveness is not a case of 'selling' the idea by urging all kinds of claims about the benefit your study will bring. Nor is it a matter of convincing the reviewers of your enthusiasm for the piece of knowledge you intend to pursue. Although these things have a place, what persuades is an argument which supports the stated purpose for the research. Good argument also instils reviewers with confidence that you know what you are talking about and might be trusted to carry out the project effectively. It allows you to demonstrate your command of the subject matter and your understanding of what is involved in the proposed research.

Being succinct

Being effective in writing grant proposals has much to do with providing enough information so as to be understood—but using as few words as possible. A fine balance is to be achieved between clarity of meaning and brevity. The key to finding the balance lies with sentence structure and choice of words. When the first draft of the document is complete, put it away for at least a week. Then re-read it with a view to removing unnecessary words, irrelevant sentences or sections that are not essential to the argument. Re-write sections if the meaning can be made clearer by using fewer words. Allow time in your planning for this editing stage of proposal development.

Completing the application form

Once the proposal has been finalised you can complete the application form. It is most important to follow instructions exactly and provide *all* the information and documentation required when completing the form. It is essential too that you type responses onto the form. Helping the granting body to read your application is a good strategy. Fit what you have to say in the space provided wherever possible. A handy hint is to make a couple of copies of the forms and use these for drafts. When you are satisfied that you have the information organised to fit the spaces—type it onto the original. You can then copy the completed original to retain as your record and destroy the drafts. The closing date for applications *must* be adhered to.

Conclusion

It is common to underestimate the work involved in writing a grant proposal. The process requires as much time, consideration and preparation as you would need to write for publication. The proposal is presented to reviewers in your place, and therefore it must speak for you. Thus it is in your interests to muster all the skills you have at your command to create a good impression through your writing.

REFERENCES

Hamilton H, Gray G 1992 A guide to successful grant applications. Royal College of
   Nursing Australia, Melbourne
Sultz H, Scherwin F 1981 Grant writing for health professionals. Little, Brown, Boston
Wilson H 1985 Research in nursing. Addison-Wesley, Menlo Park

4. Satisfying ethics committees

George Sadleir, Jeanette Robertson

The content of this chapter is intended to include a general guide to the working of ethics committees and to describe the considerations which such committees take into account in assessing and deciding upon the worth and validity of research projects. It is hoped that the information provided may not only help to acquaint intending nurse researchers with the essential ethical requirements of a research project but also give an insight into what will be expected for the approval of the project by an ethics committee.

The need for a research project to be approved by the ethics committee of an institution should not be regarded as an extraneous obstacle to be overcome: the ethical evaluation of the project is, in fact, an integral part of the process of research. Even proposed research which is seemingly of a trivial nature should be referred to the IEC (institutional ethics committee) for approval. There may also be situations in which a doubt arises as to whether a procedure or program amounts to research or, rather, comes under the heading of quality assurance, an educational exercise or innovative medical or nursing practice. Where such a doubt exists, the matter should be referred to the ethics committee. Remember, also, that the ethics committee of any particular institution is usually prepared to give guidance in advance towards compliance with its requirements and that assistance should always be sought.

ROLES, FUNCTIONS AND EXPECTATIONS

Membership and obligations

The IEC of a hospital, academic establishment or other institution whose activities involve an area of medical research has the primary duty to review and authorise or refuse requests for research proposed to be carried out within, or under the auspices of, the institution. The IEC must ensure that ethical standards are maintained in research projects to protect the interests of the research subjects, the investigator and the institution. As well as adjudicating upon research projects, the IEC will also often have the obligation to provide advice within the institution in relation to ethical policy generally or upon specific topics which arise for decision.

Membership

The membership of an IEC is usually drawn from a variety of backgrounds including not only medical, nursing and other health professionals who are employed by or attached to the institution, but also individuals from the wider community. In 1992, the National Health and Medical Research Council (NH&MRC) in Australia laid down the requirements for the composition of an IEC as follows:

(i) an IEC shall be composed of men and women of different age groups and include at least one member from each of the following categories:
- laywoman not associated with the institution
- layman not associated with the institution
- minister of religion
- lawyer
- medical graduate with research experience
(ii) persons may be appointed to stand-in for members when necessary;
(iii) an institution may appoint more persons that those specified in (i) as members of an IEC;
(iv) members and stand-in members shall be appointed by an institution on such terms and conditions as the institution determines and in such manner as to ensure that the Committee will fulfil its responsibilities;
(v) members shall be appointed as individuals for their expertise and not in a representative capacity;
(vi) a lay person is one who is not closely involved in medical, scientific or legal work.
(vii) a minister of religion may be of any faith.

In a hospital, the members of the IEC generally include the medical director and the director of nursing (or their nominees) as well as representatives from the clinical staff and from medical departments such as pathology, genetics and oncology. Allied health professionals may also be represented together with persons engaged in the field of medical and health research itself.

From outside the institution, as well as persons who are from the legal profession or the clergy, there may be members who are ethicists or from the social sciences. Other lay members will usually have a background of experience and interest in social and health issues. The experience and expertise of members from outside the institution contributes to the IEC's breadth of ethical considerations and to its appreciation of the human and social effects of particular projects.

Although representation on the IEC by persons other than health professionals is of essential importance, the assessment of scientific validity of a research project, its usefulness of purpose, the likelihood of adverse physical or psychological effects upon subjects and the competence and qualifications of researchers are obviously matters upon which advice must be contributed by those members who have the appropriate professional qualifications. In some IECs, a panel of appropriately qualified members may be delegated to make an initial assessment of a project for scientific validity before it is referred to the Committee as a whole.

Regulation of research

In Australia, IECs are given a high degree of freedom from statutory or other governmental regulation. That freedom is generally regarded as beneficial in that, without compromising the need for the rigorous ethical survey of projects under their consideration, IECs continue to retain a flexibility and informality of procedure which may be adapted to meet particular cases and which allows for expedition in the processing of applications for approval of research. The NH&MRC in its *Statement on Human Experimentation* (1992) adopted the requirements that, in carrying out its functions, an IEC shall:

(i) conform with the NH&MRC Statement and Supplementary Notes as published from time to time;
(ii) while promoting the advance of knowledge by research, ensure that the rights of the subjects of research take precedence over the expected benefits to human knowledge;
(iii) ensure that, in all projects involving human subjects and relating to health, the free and informed consent of the subjects will be obtained;
(iv) ensure that no member of the committee adjudicates on projects in which they may be personally involved;
(v) ensure that research projects take into consideration local cultural and social attitudes;
(vi) give its own consideration to projects that involve research in more than one institution;
(vii) require the principal investigator to disclose any previous decisions regarding the project made by another IEC and whether the protocol is presently before another IEC; and
(viii) determine the method of monitoring appropriate to each project.

Under the NH&MRC requirements, to achieve appropriate monitoring of research projects until their completion the IEC must:

(i) at regular periods, and not less frequently than annually, require principal investigators to provide reports on matters including:
  • security of records;
  • compliance with approved consent procedures and documentation;
  • compliance with other special conditions;

(ii) as a condition of approval of the protocol require that investigators report immediately anything which might affect ethical acceptance of the protocol, including:
  • adverse effects on subjects;
  • proposed changes in the protocol; and
  • unforeseen events that might affect continued ethical acceptability of the project.

The committee must also establish confidential mechanisms for receiving complaints or reports on the conduct of the project.

The research protocol

The protocol of a research study is the formal written statement of the project as proposed by the researcher and to be agreed upon by the subjects, the IEC and the scientific community. Its content must recognise and meet the requirements of the public interest, i.e. that:

  (i) any medical or nursing research should have the potential of beneficial results;
 (ii) the research will not harm the persons who are to be the subjects of the study; and
(iii) the investigators will regard all personal information with due respect and confidentiality.

The IEC will normally have its own set of guidelines for the preparation and structure of the protocol and the information to be presented to it upon an application for approval and you should make reference, at an early stage, to these guidelines and seek advice from the administrator or other staff of the institution who are attached to the IEC.

In its application of ethical principles, an IEC will include the relevant rules and recommendations of the NH&MRC as formulated through the Australian Health Ethics Committee of the Council.

Objectives of the research

It is trite to say that, in any proposal for research, responsibly undertaken, the investigator has a clear idea of the objective which it is hoped to achieve by the project. In this regard, your project should be directed towards answering a primary question. It is *crucial* that this question, as well as any subsidiary questions, are carefully chosen and precisely stated in your protocol.

Many experienced investigators spend a great deal of time in defining and expressing the main objective of their study. Once that clarity has been achieved, the remainder of the protocol may become a series of subsidiary steps which describe the technique for collection of the relevant information.

Using this method, you will identify for yourself, as well as for those who scrutinise the project, that the study is practicable and capable of completion. Indeed, ethical approval can only be granted if there is sufficient evidence to demonstrate the likelihood that the study is capable of satisfactory completion.

It is not enough for you to state merely a broad objective for the study, nor is it acceptable to state expectations which are too high. For example, to say that a project 'will identify' the environmental and other causes of a particular disease or condition is both optimistic and misleading—if what is really intended is an epidemiological survey to ascertain whether or not there are environmental factors which may be found commonly to recur in the sufferers from the particular disease or condition.

Again, you may have the intention by your research to test a hypothesis which you have formulated. In such a case, you should state clearly the primary question which you are seeking to answer. Protocols which list several objectives in the same general topic are open to suspicion as being 'fishing expeditions' or 'data dredging exercises.' Although this may be a useful technique for the generation of hypotheses, it should be avoided when the object is to test a hypothesis.

Background information and scientific references

In preparing the project you should demonstrate the appropriate knowledge of literature relating to previous studies in the same area. Write the protocol for those who are not familiar with the particular field of knowledge and present a logical and coherent account of the subject so that the problem which you seek to resolve or the hypothesis to be tested is presented against the context of existing knowledge.

Describe the results of any pilot studies that you have carried out, as they may well serve to convince others that you are capable of performing the type of research for which you seek the approval. In particular, you should frame the protocol so that the scientific justification for the study and its potential benefits are clear to anyone who reads it.

Study endpoints

The study endpoint is the outcome which is to be measured in order to answer the objective of the research, e.g. a study of chemotherapeutic agents might be interested in quality of life, objective response rates and survival times. You should establish a single endpoint to evaluate the principal objective of the study. If you use several, combined or alternative, endpoints the probability of a chance positive result increases. If the results are inconsistent, an explanation of the inconsistencies may be difficult and unconvincing.

During the course of your research you may find that you obtain a reliable answer to the objective of the study at an earlier stage in the program than you had anticipated. Where a study involves interventions which may cause serious side effects, it is obviously unethical to continue the program once a reliable answer has been obtained. But in any case of human research, it is unethical—and also very inefficient—to wait until the results on all persons have been obtained before drawing conclusions when a reliable result is already available.

Thus, in the course of the research you should demonstrate a flexible approach in monitoring progress with due regard for appropriate statistical techniques. In addition, all protocols for clinical trials must declare the mechanism to be applied for the completion of the study and, as appropriate, lay down criteria for early closure. Finally, you should remember that no study is better than the quality of its data. You must therefore be prepared to keep meticulous records in work books, on data sheets or on floppy disks.

Financial matters

You have an obligation to obtain or provide funding which is adequate to enable your study to be completed according to the protocol. Your protocol therefore should include full information as to the sources and extent of funding.

In the case of hospital based research, no charge may be made to a patient or imposed upon the hospital's budget for procedures beyond those involved in routine clinical care. Volunteers may be compensated for inconvenience or for loss of time but any such payment should not be so large as to amount to an inducement to take part in a research project.

Recruitment of subjects

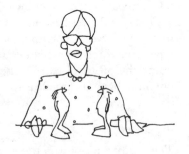

Give careful consideration to the method by which subjects are to be recruited and how they are to be approached (including information sheets and letters of invitation to participate). You will need to include that information in the protocol. Whatever method you use to approach subjects, you must always make clear to them that they are completely free to refuse to participate in the study and/or to withdraw from it without fear of retribution—even after they have agreed to take part.

If you intend that patients of a hospital are to be included as subjects, take into account their vulnerability and dependence upon the hospital and that you will be required to notify the attending consultant in advance of your intention to approach a patient. Be careful not to intrude into existing professional relationships. You may advertise for research subjects but any advertisement should contain no more than brief details of the project and of the person to be contacted. (Further information about this and other recruitment strategies may be found in Ch. 5.)

Criteria for recruitment. The criteria which you propose for the selection of subjects of your research should be precisely stated in the protocol—together with the steps which you will take to screen volunteers for their suitability.

It is not enough, for example, to say that 'patients with rheumatoid arthritis will be included in the study.' There must be a clear and, wherever possible, objective list of factors which define the criteria for inclusion. Those criteria have importance in determining the availability of subjects for recruitment into the study and, eventually, the extent to which the results of the study may come to have practical benefit and application.

Equally, you should establish unequivocal criteria for exclusion of those who are unlikely to benefit from the study (other than subjects who are recruited as controls). It may, for example, be a study in which it is necessary for you to exclude pregnant patients; in such a case the steps which you propose to take to ensure their exclusion should be documented.

Numbers to be recruited. The numbers of persons to be studied and the justification for that number must be declared in your protocol. It is unethical to choose a sample size based purely upon a set length of time, the amount of resources that are available or upon some arbitrary figure. Make sure that the study will have sufficient statistical power from which to detect differences which are of clinical interest. It is unethical to either include too few subjects to enable valid conclusions to be reached or to recruit more subjects that are needed.

Inexperienced investigators tend to exaggerate their ability to attract patients or other persons into a study. That tendency, combined with poor organisational assistance, may make it impossible to carry out or complete the study. If necessary, you should perform pilot studies in order to establish accurate grounds for the estimate of the numbers and availability of subjects required. In certain cases, it will be wise to allow for and define measures to permit the continuation of the study should unforeseen circumstances influence the recruitment rate.

Control groups and allocation of subjects

It is sound scientific practice to compare the effects of a new therapy with a control group. The random allocation of subjects to the control group and the group which is to be the subject of intervention by the research is the preferred method—as this method avoids bias.

If your study requires the allocation of subjects to groups, you should detail the procedure for randomisation and include a description of the types of patients to be entered in the study. You should also stipulate how any patients under active treatment, who are allocated into a study group destined to receive a placebo, will continue to receive what is considered to be the best treatment currently available.

'Blinding' techniques are applied in order to diminish the problems of inbuilt bias during the collection and assessment of research data. 'Single blind' studies are those in which the subject is aware of the intervention prompted by the research, but the individual carrying out the assessment of the subject does not know in whether the subject has been placed in the 'control' group or the intervention group. In 'double blind' studies however, neither the subject nor the assessor knows the category into which the subject has been placed (e.g. a drug study where the subjects in the control group have been given a placebo). If your methodology involves any blinding of the assessors, you should make this clear in your protocol.

Scientific integrity and ethical considerations

As scientific validity is essential to the ethical approval of any project, you should design the project to ensure that it will be possible to answer the questions asked. Any project that is designed so poorly that the results cannot be properly assessed will be regarded as unethical. You must also give careful consideration to the balance of likely advantage to be gained from the project as against any discomforts, risk or inconvenience involved to the subjects. Accordingly your protocol should disclose any adverse events, effects or consequences which could result from the procedures or interventions that are involved.

You must also consider any special ethical issue which relates to your project and include, in the protocol, a discussion of those issues. Information falling into this category may include reference to matters such as the intention to obtain confidential medical data without prior consent and/or whether photographs, video recordings or sound recordings of subjects are to be made.

The researchers

Your protocol must list the personnel who will carry out the project including the chief or principal researcher who will have overall responsibility for the conduct of the study. If you are an external applicant (i.e., not employed in the proposed setting), the institution which is to be involved in the research will normally also require that one of its staff members, of sufficient seniority, be associated with your project.

Consent and confidentiality

The free consent of each person to be the subject of a research study must be obtained. Generally, an IEC will have a suitable consent form which it has approved for customary use. You have the obligation to obtain consent from each person and that requires the provision of full information, at the level of comprehension which applies to the particular person, of the purpose of the study and the methods, risks, discomfort and inconveniences which may be involved. Occasionally, an IEC will dispense with the need for written consent but that will require a positive justification which you must be prepared to provide.

If your research involves visiting the home of a subject, you will need to obtain adequate permission in advance and provide proper identification at the time of contact. These and other measures which you have provided for the confidentiality of the information obtained will need to be stated in the protocol before approval can be granted to proceed by the IEC.

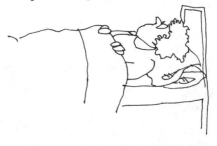

In cases where you can anticipate the proposed study is likely to occupy a lengthy period, you will need to define techniques for maintaining contact with the subjects, for example, by posting regular reports to them on progress of a study and, perhaps, making periodic contact by telephone. With appropriate permission, the details of relatives or friends of the subjects may be obtained as contacts in the event that the subjects should move from the listed address. Remember that you must always respect the right of any subject to withdraw from the project at any time.

In the publication of a research project there should be no particular identification of any individual subject and this should be stated in the protocol. It is also important for you to emphasise to the subject the measures which will apply to ensure confidentiality of the information obtained during the study.

Should your project require the inspection of existing medical records to identify those who meet the selection criteria in advance of contact with patients or subjects, you will need to demonstrate that full confidentiality will be observed. The agreement of a hospital to the provision of records will also depend upon the extent to which the provision of records will place demands upon the hospital's resources in that respect. Access to such records will normally be limited to appropriately qualified investigators and associates who are responsible to them.

In the case of subjects who are patients, the consent of the treating medical personnel is also normally required. During the course of your project, you may obtain information relating to the clinical care or well-being of a patient. In those circumstances, you have an overriding ethical duty to act in the interests of the subject even though it may prejudice the outcome and/or subsequent value of your research.

Questionnaires

The use of questionnaires to be answered by the subjects of a research project is sometimes essential. Questionnaires are however always the subject of close scrutiny by an IEC. This is because of the issue of confidentiality and the potential of the questionnaire to invade a subject's privacy through the collection of sensitive information which may even be of an incriminating nature to the subject (e.g. the use of prohibited drugs such as cannabis, amphetamines, etc.). Unless you construct the questionnaire with great care, the information provided in response to it may in any event be misleading or inadequate to achieve the results which you intend.

For these reasons, the IEC will require to see a copy of your questionnaire and of any documents which may accompany it, such as letters of introduction or information sheets. If you intend to make a direct approach to subjects with a view to completion of the questionnaire, the IEC will need to be satisfied that the method of approach is appropriate and will be made by a suitable member of the research team.

Submission of the protocol

Once you have thoroughly considered, and are in a position to meet the ethical considerations which apply to your project, you will be required to lodge the protocol and the relevant accompanying documents with the office of the IEC.

In the case of lengthy documentation, an abbreviated form of the protocol, with copies of such documents as the information sheet, consent form, questionnaire, etc., will be circulated to the members of the IEC. Should the protocol be of a lengthy nature, it is prudent for you to provide a precis with a view to giving a concise account of the project to the members of the committee.

If you are the principal investigator, you or a senior member of your research team, will usually be required to attend a meeting of the IEC before approval to the project is given. A well prepared protocol will, however, usually have served to provide the answers to the ethical requirements which members of the IEC will apply in their assessment of the project.

Content of the submission

In summary, the principal matters to be addressed in the research protocol include:

(i) background information including the scientific justification for performing the study, and the results of any pilot studies which you have carried out;

(ii) whether you have submitted the protocol to the IEC of any other institution;

(iii) a concise account of the objectives of your study and its endpoints;
(iv) the criteria for inclusion and exclusion of subjects;
 (v) the method by which you intend to recruit subjects, including reference to advertising for volunteers, the use of subjects who are in situations of dependence (such as hospital patients) and procedures to avoid interference with existing professional relationships;
(vi) the basis on which you have ascertained the numbers of subjects which you require (sample size) and the mechanisms which you intend to apply for the prolongation of the study (should that become necessary) and its closure; and
(vii) a detailed description of the study design and techniques with copies of such documents as draft questionnaires, letters of invitation to subjects, information sheets and consent forms.

Misconduct in research

An IEC has the responsibility to maintain vigilance to ensure as far as possible that the approved research is carried out ethically and there is no incident of misconduct in its execution. There have been recent examples of such misconduct occurring, even on the part of prominent and experienced researchers. These episodes have emphasised the need for IECs to monitor closely the progress of experiments, and to listen to members of staff who may raise problems after a study has begun. In an effort to increase the awareness of researchers of their ethical and professional responsibilities when undertaking research, the University of Western Australia has developed guidelines on research ethics and misconduct for use by researchers. As these guidelines were intended and approved for use within that university, they have not been widely publicised. The following list, consonant with the University of Western Australia's guidelines relates to clinical nursing research.

Guidelines on research ethics and misconduct

According to the University of Western Australia guidelines, misconduct in research may be identified by any of the following characteristics:

 (i) the fabrication of data, claiming results where none has been obtained;*
(ii) the falsification of data, including changing records;
(iii) plagiarism, including the direct copying of textual material, the use of other people's data without acknowledgment, and the use of ideas from other people without adequate attribution;

---

* Unintentional misinterpretation of data does not constitute misconduct.

(iv) misleading ascription of authorship, including the listing of authors without their permission and attributing work to others who have not in fact contributed to the research, and the lack of appropriate acknowledgment of work primarily reduced by a research student/ trainee or associate;

(v) other practices that seriously deviate from those commonly accepted within the research community for proposing, conducting or reporting research;

(vi) intimidation of a research worker, and/or bringing undue pressure to bear by one research worker upon another, to misrepresent results and/or authorship; and

(vii) conducting spurious research on behalf of a sponsor organisation, e.g. purely to gain tax offset benefits;

(viii) conduct contrary to ethics guidelines.

The chairperson of an IEC will accept, and regard as confidential, any concerns raised about misconduct in research. If it is considered appropriate, the matter will be reported to other authorities and to the board of management of the institution.

PRACTICAL STRATEGIES TO SECURE APPROVAL

By now you will have probably realised that the sub-mission of a protocol to an IEC is a systematic process which requires you to provide specific details about your study to a formally constituted committee. As outlined in the first part of this chapter, IECs exist not only to protect the rights of the study subjects, but also to ensure that any research undertaken within the organisation has the potential to yield valid, reliable, *useful* results.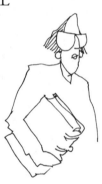

When seeking approval from your nominated institu-tion to undertake your research, you will have at least one opportunity to convince the agency's IEC as to the value of your research project—through the submission of your research protocol. In addition, where human subjects are required for the study (as opposed to a review of case notes), you may also be called before the IEC to explain your research in more detail, and to answer any questions the members of the committee may have about the conduct of your study.

Apart from the documentary requirements already discussed however, there are also a number of procedural tasks associated with the submission of a research protocol which can facilitate the process. While the completion of these tasks in themselves cannot guarantee the committee's sanction, working through the stages described below should enhance the chances of obtaining approval to undertake your study in your chosen setting.

Visit the proposed setting

It is in your best interest to visit each agency you plan to use *prior* to submitting your protocol. The purpose of this visit is to discuss the possibility of implementing your study in your chosen setting and ensure that all the requirements of your research design can be fulfilled in the time allocated to the conduct of the study. Chapter 5 outlines the factors which should be considered when assessing a potential research setting and you should refer to this chapter for further information about this integral part of the research process.

Obtain the relevant guidelines

Obtain the institution's guidelines for the conduct of research. While the basic requirements for the content of research protocols seldom differ from those described earlier in this chapter, IECs sometimes require additional information about the conduct of a study before they will consider approving the proposed research. To enhance an applicant's chances of meeting both the ordinary and the specific requirements, IECs normally provide guidelines which specify the required format and content for protocols submitted to their institution for consideration. You should obtain a copy of these regulations during your initial visit to your chosen setting. Furthermore, as the specific requirements may vary between institutions, if you plan to collect your data from more than one setting, you will need to acquire a copy of the requirements of each IEC to direct you in your preparation.

Obtain university approval to commence your study

If you are undertaking your research as part of the requirements for a higher degree, as soon as you have confirmed the suitability of your chosen venue, your initial step should be to obtain approval for your research from the IEC at your university. Even though you may obtain approval from the university however, you should be aware that this will not include automatic access to your study population. As such, you will still be required to convince the IEC in the research setting that your study is of sufficient merit to warrant approval for its conduct.

IECs in hospitals and health care agencies usually require evidence that the protocols submitted by students have been approved by the appropriate university research and ethics committees before they will consider giving permission for the conduct of a study. The advantage of this is that problems which may jeopardise your protocol's chances of approval can be identified and remedied before they are considered by the IEC in the hospital or health care agency. Therefore, it is only when you have obtained the approval of the IEC at your university to proceed with your study, that you should consider submitting your protocol to the IEC in the research setting.

Comply with guidelines

As meetings of IECs are normally held monthly, approval to conduct research can often take several weeks to obtain. It is therefore in your interest to submit your protocol as soon as you have all the necessary information that you need to satisfy the institution's requirements. On no account however, should you *sacrifice* the content (or presentation) of your submission in order to satisfy a meeting deadline. It may mean that your protocol will not contain sufficient information to allow the committee to make a decision as to the value, feasibility and/or integrity of your research.

When preparing your protocol, it is essential that you follow the institution's guidelines *to the letter*. If you are planning to use more than one setting, this may mean that you will have to produce a slightly different document to suit the requirements of each agency. It is in your interests to do this however, as failure to comply with the stated specifications may result in a request for amendments to your protocol, and a delay in commencing your study while you revise your submission to conform with their requirements.

Notwithstanding the conditions specified in the guidelines, if your methodology calls for the study of subjects who will be unable to give informed consent, e.g. children, or demented or psychotic patients, you will need to stipulate the conditions for their inclusion in the study. If you are seeking approval to use direct observation of these groups to collect your data, you will need to discuss the risks, benefits and the ethical implications of your research in some detail. In particular, you will need to demonstrate to the IEC that the value of observing the subjects without their permission clearly outweighs the need to obtain their informed consent. Failure to address these and other significant issues adequately may result in the outright rejection of your submission or, at best, intensive questioning at the IEC meeting.

Review the documentation

Before you submit your protocol, read it through carefully. As you read it, be sure that you can adequately explain and/or justify every aspect of the content. The IEC will expect you to be very familiar with all elements of the proposed study. Committee members are not to know which points you have not fully come to terms with, and consequently may ask you questions which you may find very difficult to answer at the meeting. If you can't explain a point, obtain the information which will allow you to do so before submitting your protocol. Do not be tempted to leave out all the points that you cannot either justify or adequately explain as this strategy will not necessarily solve your problem. If the information you omit is essential to obtaining IEC approval, (e.g. how you will go about obtaining consent) you can still expect to be questioned about the subject when you attend the meeting.

Institutional ethics committee meetings

If you are required to attend an IEC meeting, you can expect to receive notification as to the time and place of the meeting from the committee secretariat following the submission of your protocol. As IEC meetings may deal with several submissions and a variety of other business, you will be required to attend only that part of the meeting which relates to the discussion of your protocol.

When you receive notification of the meeting, don't panic. Would be researchers who go to IEC meetings with scientifically sound research protocols which address relevant questions, who know how they are going to conduct their studies, and who are mindful of the rights of their potential subjects, seldom have difficulties at IEC meetings. Indeed, some researchers have even been known to have enjoyed the challenge of defending their protocols.

If you are a student or an external applicant, it is customary for the committee to request that your supervisor or the principal researcher accompany you to the meeting. Apart from providing you with some moral support, the presence of an experienced researcher is usually requested in case some aspect of your proposed research methodology needs an explanation which is beyond your level of experience. In this regard, it will be in your interests to ensure your supervisor has a copy of your submission before you attend the meeting.

Preparing for the meeting

Some preparation is called for before you attend an IEC meeting. As some weeks may elapse between submitting your protocol and being called upon to defend it, there is a chance you may forget some of the fine detail it contains. Applicants who look vague about the content of their protocols, tend to give the members of the committee a negative impression of their competence, and therefore their ability to undertake the study. Therefore, the greatest favour you can do for yourself prior to facing the IEC is to ensure that you are thoroughly conversant with the contents of your protocol.

As you revise the content of your submission, think about how you can justify the need for your research, and what impact it will ultimately have on practice. In this regard you should have a good grasp of the relevant literature, so that you can be ready to explain how your study will create new knowledge (or confirm previous findings) if you are asked to elaborate on its value. You should also be able to explain, in terms the lay persons on the committee will be able to understand, the proposed changes to practice, and any risks which may be associated with the change. Furthermore, you may like to consider the consequences for clinical practice if the problem being researched is not investigated.

In addition to a detailed knowledge of the protocol's content, the committee will expect you to have given some thought to the practical aspects of conducting your study, e.g. how you will go about selecting and recruiting your sample (in and outside regular working hours), and how you plan to manage the collection of your data. The committee may also wish to ascertain how your study will impact on the regular work load of the staff and the resources of the setting.

If you are not employed in your chosen agency, you may need to make an appointment to return to the setting before you meet with the committee. The purpose of this visit is to confirm that your expectations about conducting the study are not unrealistic. While it remains a sad fact of life that some protocols are rejected by IECs because there is insufficient information provided in the submission to enable an accurate assessment of the impact of the study on the setting to be made, others fail because the stated arrangements for recruitment and data collection seem to be incongruent with the proposed setting. You can guard against the latter possibility by addressing the feasibility in the setting of your proposed methods in your protocol, and being prepared to elaborate this important aspect of your study at the meeting.

Winning approval at the meeting

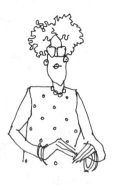

While you should be fully conversant with the content of your protocol, take a copy along to the meeting in case the need arises to refer to it during the course of your interview. When you are called into the meeting, expect to see a committee of some 10–12 people. All of them will be expecting you to demonstrate that you have the competence to undertake successfully the study you have proposed. It is up to you to convince them that you can do just that.

Commonly (although not always), the first request is for an applicant to describe the proposed study briefly. Here a *concise* statement of the problem, the proposed method and what you hope to achieve is called for. If you have done your homework this request will be relatively easy to satisfy, as the basic principles underlying your study will be fresh and clear in your mind. If you are unsure how much detail is required, err on the side of brevity. The committee will ask for more information should it be required. Don't make the mistake of launching into a rambling discourse on your pet subject. You may inadvertently make some broad general statements which you may find difficult to substantiate later on.

Once you have provided an overview of your study, questions will usually be directed towards clarifying specific aspects of your proposed methodology. If you don't hear the question properly (or understand it), ask to have it repeated or clarified. This is important as, if you miss the point, the committee may be denied vital information which they may need to approve your study. The presence of your supervisor may come in useful here. An experienced ear often can discern exactly what is being asked and come up with the right answer on your behalf. It may therefore be prudent to seek the assistance from your ally when coping with questions which are outside your knowledge and expertise. Don't use this tactic too often though, it will undermine the committee's perception of your ability to conduct your research independently.

Once the committee has obtained the required information you will be excused from the meeting. Do not expect to get a decision regarding approval (or otherwise) immediately. It is not until you have left the meeting that the committee will discuss your submission and decide whether your protocol should be approved, revised, amended or rejected. It is usual that applicants are advised of the committee's decision by mail as soon as possible after the meeting.

Conclusion

While gaining the approval of the institutional ethics committee in your chosen setting may be seen to be a time consuming and somewhat tedious task, it is an essential component of any research project which requires the use of human subjects. In this chapter we have presented information which we hope will assist you to meet the requirements of the IEC in your chosen setting. While the specific requirements of institutions may vary in accordance with their role, and clientele, the underlying principles, which address the rights and protection of persons asked to participate as subjects in research, are essentially similar for all health care agencies. It is the satisfaction of these general principles that have been addressed in these pages.

NOTE

In preparing the information in this chapter, we wish to acknowledge the substantial contribution of information from the policies and guidelines in use by the Ethics Committee of Royal Perth Hospital. Those policies and guidelines have also been adapted for use in modified form at the Princess Margaret Hospital for Children in Perth.

We are also grateful to Dr Peter D. Sly MD FRACP, Head of the Division of Clinical Sciences at the WA Research Institute for Child Health, for his contribution to the content of this chapter and to the Research Committee, University of Western Australia for its permission to draw from their Guidelines for Research Ethics and Misconduct.

REFERENCES

Ethics Committee, Royal Perth Hospital 1991 Operating policies and guidelines.
National Health & Medical Research Foundation 1987 Statement on human
   experimentation. Dept Community Services & Health, Canberra

5. Planning and conducting research

Western Australian Nurse Researchers' Network

Undertaking research in a hospital or health care agency can be an extremely rewarding experience. The successful completion of a clinical project does not however come as a matter of luck. It results from careful planning and organisation which are the keys to the conduct of trouble free clinical research. This chapter describes those factors which should be considered during the planning, implementation and conduct of research in the clinical setting. All have been found by nurse researchers to influence the outcome of clinical studies. The assumption has been made that when the organisation and administration of the study is sound, the likelihood of problems arising will be minimised. Consequently the discussion related to the difficulties which may be encountered during the course of clinically based research has been reserved until Chapter 6.

Selecting a research setting

The selection of an appropriate setting is crucial to the success of your study. It is our experience that the outcome of any clinical nursing research is directly dependent on:

- relevance of the research problem to the chosen setting;
- feasibility of conducting the planned research in the chosen setting;
- calibre of the instruments/research assistants used to collect the data; and
- success of the strategies used to implement and conduct the study.

Relevance of the problem to the setting

During the conduct of our studies we have found that co-operation by nurses working in the research setting is maximal when they can:

- see the relevance of the research problem to their own work practices;
- expect the findings of the study to improve their nursing care.

In these cases we have found that staff are far more likely to co-operate with the tasks associated with the collection of data than if irrelevant questions are imposed upon them by an outside source. You should bear this in mind when considering a setting for your study.

Assessing the feasibility of a setting

Visit the setting

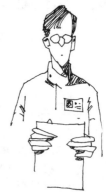

Once you have decided upon a potential location for your study, you should organise a visit to assess its suitability as a research setting. Your visit will enable you to both confirm that all the requirements of your methodology can be fulfilled, and identify any factors which may influence the implementation of your study. If you already work in the setting, it is likely that these conditions will already be known to you. If you are external to the institution, reconnaissance is absolutely essential *before* you submit your proposal for approval by the institutional ethics committee (IEC).

To arrange your visit, contact the director of nursing or nominated research co-ordinator at the hospital or agency you wish to access to discuss your study. If a change to practice is planned, negotiate an appointment time to observe the current practice so that you can ascertain how your proposed intervention might be implemented. To facilitate future contact, request the name of a liaison person who can answer any questions you may have about gaining approval to undertake your study and its implementation following approval by the IEC.

Factors influencing the conduct of the study

Availability of subjects. During your visit, observe all the areas where you hope to undertake your research. Check that it will be possible to implement your proposed recruitment strategies and also that the potential exists for you to recruit at least twice your required sample size in the time available to you. Many factors such as ward closures, public holidays, medical conferences and the influence of the seasons on shift workers and on certain medical conditions (e.g. asthma) have the potential to reduce recruitment opportunities. You will therefore need to consider these factors when estimating recruitment time and assessing the ability of the setting to provide the necessary numbers of study subjects.

Restrictions on access to subjects. In addition to the environmental and seasonal factors which may limit the availability of potential subjects, agencies may impose their own access restrictions on highly sought-after groups to protect them from being over researched. It is therefore important to check whether your proposed study population will be subject to such restrictions. *Never* simply assume that subjects will be available for your research just because sufficient numbers of people fitting the inclusion criteria for your study exist in the setting.

Impact on work load. If you plan to rely on the staff to collect data for you, the impact of your research on their work load will also need to be carefully considered. This is particularly important if other studies or ward projects are already in progress. For the reasons outlined in Chapter 6, staff who collect data for other people's projects do not always see the potential benefits of the information they collect. In practice this means that where two studies are running concurrently, there is always a chance that nurses or subjects will be less conscientious about providing data for a complex study than for one which requires considerably less effort—regardless of its origin or the potential of the findings to improve practice. From a nurse's point of view, the best kind of research does not add substantially to the work load. Remember this as you assess the impact of your project in the proposed setting, and if possible, avoid those settings where studies are already in progress.

Availability of equipment or consumable items. When assessing a setting for a study which requires the use of equipment, you should check that any instrument/s required will be available for your use during data collection. If the use of consumable items will be required, (e.g. dressing packs, swab sticks, syringes etc.) it will facilitate the conduct of the study if the items are already part of the usual stock. While this condition is not an absolute prerequisite for a research setting, it does simplify the processes associated with the supply and reimbursement of materials used during the collection of data.

It is only after you have confirmed that it is feasible to conduct your study in your chosen setting within the time available to you, that you can be confident that the study has a good chance of being successfully completed. Therefore it is not until this stage that you can finalise your research protocol and submit it to the IEC for approval.

Choosing a valid data collection instrument

The means by which you choose to collect your data, i.e. your data collection instrument, can take many forms. While the questionnaire is possibly the most common of all data collection instruments, observation charts, (e.g. for monitoring vital signs or fluid balance) or assessment charts, (e.g. for evaluating pain or wound healing) may also be used for the purpose. While the nature of your study will normally dictate the type of instrument you should use, the options open to you to obtain a suitable means of collecting your data are essentially the same whether your design is experimental or descriptive. Essentially you have the choice between:

- using a pre-existing instrument in its original form;
- modifying a pre-existing instrument to suit local conditions; or
- developing and validating a new instrument for your own use.

Using a pre-existing instrument

If you are planning to replicate a previous study to ascertain whether similar findings can be obtained in your setting using the same methodology, you will need to obtain the original data collection instrument—if a direct comparison of results at the completion of your study is to be possible. It is both bad practice and bad manners to use someone else's instrument without his or her permission. While it can be argued that, once published, data collection tools become a matter of public record, using an instrument as it appears in a journal article may lead to problems in the conduct of the research. This is because authors sometimes withhold vital information from publication, such as keys to interpretation, to guard against the unauthorised use of the tool. For this reason, you will need to request a copy of the complete instrument together with permission to use it from its developer or the copyright holder before you attempt to replicate the study.

Although permission to use an instrument is usually relatively easy to obtain, some conditions may be placed on its use for research. Write to the author at the address stated in the research article. If the article is more than two years old, check the recent nursing indexes (described in Ch. 2) for a more recent reference to the author to confirm or update the address.

In your letter to the author, specify the details of your proposed project and how you plan to use the instrument. Request a reply by a specified date, and if you have not received a reply by your deadline, consider telephoning the agency (i.e. university or hospital) to confirm the address is correct. In the absence of a reply from the author, the journal editor may be able to help you with a current address or (if the journal holds the copyright) grant permission to use the tool. Permission from this source, however, will not guarantee that you have the entire instrument. In these cases it will be up to you to decide whether to proceed without the original data collection instrument.

Modifying an existing instrument

Whilst using another researcher's method as the basis for your own data collection tool may save you considerable time during the development of your proposal, the decision to modify a pre existing instrument should not be made lightly. Ultimately it will limit your ability to make direct comparisons with the findings of the original study. Data obtained using the modified version of an instrument should however enable you to compare the trends which emerge from your data with those arising from the original research, as well as providing the specific information which will answer your research question.

Before you decide to modify an existing instrument, consider the characteristics of the study population for which it was originally designed. A questionnaire or other data collection instrument/s developed for use with specific socioeconomic, cultural or age groups cannot normally be modified for use by groups other than those for which it was developed. This is because:

- if the original questions incorporated vernacular or figurative language, their meaning will be lost or at least distorted during a literal translation of the words;
- if questions were directed at the values or beliefs of a specific culture or class, they may be misinterpreted by individuals who are not familiar with them; and
- skills possessed by adults (e.g. discrimination) are not always present in children, or even adolescents. Likewise the problem solving abilities present in many young adults may no longer be present in elderly subjects.

For these reasons, if you do elect to modify an existing instrument, choose one that was developed for a study population similar to your own.

Substitution is the most common means of modification. For example, language may be modified to reflect local usage (e.g. Pethidine for Meperidine, nappy for diaper). Where measures of physiological function are required, it may be possible to use alternative equipment (e.g. mercury for electronic thermometers, sphygmomanometers for Dinamap machines) without jeopardising the validity of the data.

Be aware that the modification of questionnaires designed to measure concepts is not recommended for the novice. Even seemingly minor changes to the content may undermine the validity of the tool, (i.e. its ability to measure what it is supposed to measure) and consequently jeopardise the quality of the data.

If you change an instrument, it is imperative that a pilot study be undertaken to check its validity and the quality of the data arising from its use. If this can be established, modifying an existing instrument will eliminate the lengthy process of developing and establishing the intrinsic validity of a new tool. It is recommended, however, that you seek the advice of experts if you are contemplating instrument modification.

Developing a data collection instrument

For original research questions where suitable data collection instruments are not already available, you will need to develop and validate your own tool. This is a difficult and time consuming option, but essential if your question is addressing a unique problem.

Before you start designing your own instrument, you must be certain about what you want to achieve by using it. If you are a novice researcher, you would be well advised to seek assistance from both a content specialist and someone skilled in the development of data collection instruments.

Content. A 'content specialist' is someone with extensive knowledge of the subject area under investigation. Clinical nurse specialists/consultants often make ideal content specialists. While these practitioners may not necessarily be experienced in the conduct of research, they can usually be of valuable assistance in determining the content of your questionnaire or assessment tool. They may also be able to identify confounding variables and/or limitations of the sample or setting which may impinge upon the content of your data collection instrument. It will therefore be to your advantage to find a specialist to assist you with this aspect of your research design.

Validity and reliability. Deciding upon the content is but one aspect of the development process. The instrument must be capable of yielding the valid and reliable data which will enable you to answer your research question, in a form which is compatible with your proposed method of data analysis.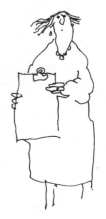

There are many types of validity, ranging from the primitive face validity through to the more complex construct and predictive forms. While it is not necessary to establish all types of validity for your data collection instrument, it is imperative that you confirm that your tool is a valid measure of the variable or concept under investigation before you attempt to implement your study. In their book *Measurement in Nursing Research,* Waltz, Strickland and Lenz (1991) describe the various forms of validity in detail. It is recommended as a useful source of information regarding the process of instrument validation.

Statistical advice. If you require any advice about the analysis of your data, you should seek it early, preferably when you have completed the first draft of your data collection instrument and are at the stage of compiling your research proposal. *Under no circumstances* should you defer seeking statistical advice until after you have finished collecting your data. By then it is too late to rectify any flaws in the research design which may have jeopardised its validity. While biostatisticians are the preferred consultants for nursing research, if you do not have access to such a specialist, any researcher with experience in data analysis may be able to assist you.

When seeking advice about data analysis, try to visit the proposed research setting with the statistician. This will set your study in context and illustrate what you are trying to achieve. As an indication of the statistician's understanding of your requirements, request a written statement which not only describes the most appropriate method of analysing your data, but also demonstrates an understanding of the problem being studied. It is often a good idea to incorporate this statement into the proposal you submit for IEC approval as evidence of co-opted expertise.

Research assistants

For studies which incorporate observation or interviews in a number of locations and/or where data needs to be collected over a twenty four hour period, or seven days of the week, you will probably require assistance to conduct your research. Although adding to the cost of the study, the recruitment of assistance will make it possible for data to be collected in several places at once. However, it will also mean that you will need to address the possibility of an unchecked bias manifesting itself in the final results and establish interrater reliability before you begin data collection.

Recruiting research assistants

Before you appoint any research assistant, consider whether:

- any specific skills are required to perform the required tasks. The nature of the research methodology will normally dictate the type of skills required. For example, if data is to be collected by interview, a high level of interpersonal skills will be required.
- a knowledge of nursing is essential to the data collection process (i.e. a nurse is required);
- there is a possibility that a knowledge of nursing may bias the perception of the data collector (i.e. it is not desirable to employ a nurse);
- the nature of the data to be collected cannot be influenced by a knowledge of nursing or compromised by a lack of such knowledge (i.e. a knowledge of nursing is irrelevant to the collection of the required data and a nurse or a non-nurse would be equally suitable).

Although nurses are often used to collect data for nursing research projects, they are sometimes not the best persons for the job because of the potential for bias they may bring with them to the research setting. In non-clinically based studies, or where the data collection phase does not require a knowledge of nursing, (e.g. for the assessment of patient satisfaction) consider using someone who is not a nurse and look to the employment agencies in the tertiary institutions to find an assistant. Postgraduate students looking to supplement their income are a good source of competent data collectors for projects where a knowledge of nursing is neither required nor desired, and to their advantage, are not as expensive to employ as an experienced nurse.

If you are undertaking clinical nursing research which will require the research assistant to provide some aspect of patient care, you will need to recruit a registered nurse with the appropriate level of expertise. This is because the legislation which governs the practice of nursing usually requires nursing tasks to be performed by people with an officially recognised level of nursing knowledge and skills. It is also likely that managers in the research setting will insist that registered nurses provide any nursing care which may be required.

Given that the outcome of your research will depend on the quality of the data collected, choose your research assistant carefully. Data which is incomplete, superficial, inaccurately measured, or incorrectly recorded may jeopardise the outcome of your research. Therefore when choosing an assistant, look for a person who:

* is experienced in the tasks required;
* has a background (or at least an interest) in the subject of your research;
* is conscientious and tactful;
* pays attention to detail;
* has an understanding of the rights of research subjects; and
* is skilled in recognising non-verbal cues which are indicative of a subject's desire to withdraw from a study.

When recruiting an assistant, explain all the requirements of the data collection process at the time of interview, i.e. the duties involved, the hours of work (including any out of hours commitments), rates of pay, aspects of confidentiality and the proposed duration of the study. At this time it is also useful to decide upon the status of the research assistant (e.g. co-researcher, technical officer, assistant etc.) and the level of contribution which will be required to maintain that status. Your research assistant may seek recognition as co-researcher or co-author and this is a reasonable request where his or her contribution will be either significant and/or unique (as in the case of a biostatistician who may offer you the means to interpret a maze of figures, which are often generated during a complex statistical analysis).

If possible when recruiting, select only those individuals who will be available for the entire data collection period. This will eliminate the problem of having to re-establish interrater reliability once the study has commenced.

Establishing interrater reliability

Where more than one person is required to collect data using the same instrument, you will need to establish an acceptable level of interrater reliability between observers *before* you begin collecting data. While the research design can stipulate what is to be measured and the type of data which needs to be collected, it cannot anticipate how the variables being measured will be interpreted by the data collectors, or how much variability between observers can be tolerated before the reliability (and therefore the validity) of the data is jeopardised. It is therefore essential that you consider each of the risks to the validity of your data during the development of your research protocol and address each of these in turn during the training of your data collectors.

Once you have appointed your assistant/s, training should begin in order to establish consistency of data collection between data collectors. While it may be easier to work with a small number of individuals, it still may take considerable time to achieve congruity of thought between them. Therefore the sooner you can begin training, the better.

If you need statistical advice about the required level of agreement or interrater reliability, seek it at the commencement of the training program. Valid data may be useless if it is not reliable and the end of the data collection phase is too late to rectify problems related to inconsistency between data collectors.

Although watching videos specially made for training purposes is a useful way of establishing interrater reliability for studies which require the interpretation of observations or responses, videos are expensive and time-consuming to make. This type of training is therefore normally reserved for large scale studies involving several observers. Where the preparation of this type of training aid is not feasible, or where only one other person is to be involved in the collection of data, the preparation of assessment criteria or keys to interpretation of behaviour or clinical signs should be developed. These guidelines, together with training visits to the area where the research is to be undertaken will usually suffice. If you use this method however, be sure to obtain the informed consent of the people you examine, observe or survey *prior* to implementing the training process.

The training of interviewers for qualitative studies requires the implementation of more complex strategies which fall outside the scope of this book. If your study entails more than one person gathering data by interview consult Field and Morse's *Nursing Research: the Application of Qualitative Approaches* (1992) for further guidance.

Pilot studies

Once you have established the appropriate form of validity of your questionnaire or other data collection instrument and completed the preliminary training of your research assistant/s, you should arrange to conduct a pilot study in the research setting. According to Van Ort (1981),

> pilot studies are an *essential* part of the research process, in that they:
> * test the feasibility of the proposed methodology;
> * identify problems in the research design;
> * test the data collection tool for validity, reliability, sensitivity, (specificity) and objectivity;
> * allow the data collectors to gain experience dealing with the data collection instrument and the type of people who will ultimately comprise the study population.

In addition to these benefits, a pilot study will also allow you to test the feasibility of your proposed recruitment strategies and assess the rate at which you can expect to recruit your subjects.

Piloting descriptive studies

As the pilot should replicate the full scale study as closely as possible, you should select subjects in the research setting who fulfil the requirements for inclusion in your study population. Regardless of the fact that it is a pilot study, you will still need to obtain the informed consent of all participants, using the recruitment strategies described later in this chapter. This requirement is to your advantage, however, as not only will it provide an opportunity for you to identify any errors or omissions in the consent form, but it will also allow you to assess your proposed recruitment strategies. Like all recruitment exercises, when approaching people to participate in a pilot study, you should explain the nature and purpose of the study. In addition however, because it is a only trial run, you must also explain that the data they provide will not be used in the final analysis.

It is worth noting that data obtained during a pilot study is not normally included as part of the research results. Rare exceptions to this rule are when the pilot study finds no indications for change in the methodology or data collection instrument, or if the population sample is limited and/or difficult to access.

If for some reason it is not possible to undertake your pilot study in the research setting, you will need to conduct two pilot studies using two separate groups of subjects. One group should be comprised of individuals who can critically analyse your questionnaire from a format and content perspective, while the other should consist of randomly chosen individuals who can assess how easy it is to comprehend your questions and complete the form.

Piloting clinical research studies

There are many ways of inadvertently overlooking confounding variables during the planning of clinical trials, and therefore those likely to influence the data collection process must be recognised and eliminated, or controlled for, in a pilot study. To facilitate the identification of potential pitfalls in your chosen method, you should conduct a pilot study exactly as stipulated in your proposal. This is because it is only by testing the proposed process in the field that you will be able to identify any confounding variables, and/or assess how those variables that cannot be controlled will impact on the validity of he data.

A pilot study in the clinical setting will also enable you to detect any differences in interpretation which may exist between individuals observing the same phenomenon. For example, it is not until you trial the data collection techniques in the clinical setting that you can be certain that all data collectors can

- administer the specified treatment or intervention in a similar manner (e.g. a pressure bandage which yields the prescribed amount of pressure on the limb of all study subjects, no matter who applies it);

- report the same clinical findings for a given set of signs (e.g. use the same clinical signs to assess the return of the gag reflex following a general anaesthetic); or
- agree on the criteria which signify a difference in an observation (e.g. between facial distortion and a facial grimace, or a pleasant expression and a smile).

As consistency of observations may vary during long studies, you should aim to establish and maintain consistency of observation in, as well as between, data collectors.

Evaluation of the pilot study

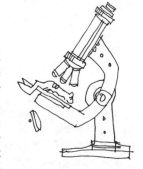

Upon completion of the pilot study, you should evaluate both the method of data collection, and the validity and reliability of the data, to identify any problems which may jeopardise the full scale study. By the time the pilot study has been completed, data collectors should have attained the predetermined level of interrater reliability. If this is not achieved, further education or training is indicated—after a reassessment of the training program which may have been deficient in the areas where the greatest discrepancies are identified.

If you are using a questionnaire to collect the data, examine the forms to detect questions which are not being answered (i.e. yielding missing values) or those which are consistently being misinterpreted. These questions may require modification or even deletion. Where computer analysis will be required, you should also check with the computing centre to ensure that the data arising from the trial are suitable for coding (see Ch. 7 for further information regarding these topics).

In some cases you may find the tool you have developed or modified is not suited to the research design. In this case you will need to decide whether the original tool is amenable to modification, or whether an alternative should be sought. If you are unsure as to the capacity of your instrument, seek the assistance of your supervisor or another experienced researcher to advise you.

Where problems or differences are identified, it is essential that you rectify the cause and repeat the piloting process until the issue is resolved. Although this may result in a number of extra trials and frustrating delays, it is *absolutely essential* that you ensure the appropriateness of your tool and/or eliminate any known problems *before* you attempt to implement your study. Ultimately you will find the time spent resolving or minimising the problems identified during the pilot study is well worth the extra effort entailed.

If you find you cannot overcome, control (or even influence) the problems identified your pilot study, look again at your reasons for wanting to conduct the research. It is unethical to collect data which has no chance of being valid, or to carry out studies which have no chance of being useful. If your study falls into either of these categories, you may need to think again about its feasibility in terms of its prospects for improving patient care. Contact your IEC for guidance if you have doubts about the study's prospects after the pilot study has been completed.

Recruiting study subjects

The key to successful recruitment is to start earlier rather than later. Due to factors foreseen and unforeseeable, gaining the required sample always takes longer than anticipated. Therefore, the sooner you can begin identifying your subjects, the better.

For samples which require specific socioeconomic or ethnic groups, you may find the Australia Post publication of direct mail lists, *List of Lists* 1993, useful. Available in paperback or on diskette, this handy reference lists the holders of mailing lists for more than 1000 occupations and ethnic groups, thereby facilitating access by potential researchers. The list may be obtained through your local Post Office for a cost of approximately thirty dollars.

Your proposal will nominate who is to make up the study population. The characteristics of the research setting will dictate how recruitment occurs. This is because the strategies required to successfully recruit healthy adults, other nurses, the intellectually handicapped, children, psychiatric patients or those with acute or life threatening illnesses are all different. You will therefore need to ensure the methods you use are appropriate for the target population.

Recruiting nurses as subjects

If your research is to be undertaken in a hospital or similar health care setting, it is often useful to make yourself known to the staff who are responsible in the course of their work for the nurses comprising the study population. They may be willing to assist you in the identification and/or selection of your sample. Such help may be in the form of:

- an offer to select a random sample for you if you are not aware of the bias of rosters and other convenient staff lists; or
- flagging members of the study population whose personal circumstances may influence their successful participation in the study.

Due to the subtle control factors which operate in a hierarchical system such as nursing, and the fact that total anonymity cannot always be guaranteed for respondents, conducting research using work colleagues as subjects is often fraught with difficulty. This is because a researcher who has seniority over members of study population is (rightly or wrongly) likely to be regarded as having the power to coerce people to participate in the study, and therefore consent may be given because of the respondent's fear of reprisals in the workplace.

The implications for this situation are that if you intend using peers and colleagues in your study, you will need to demonstrate that you can be trusted to maintain confidentiality. This can be achieved by ensuring that all ethical issues relating to anonymity and confidentiality are adequately addressed in both your proposal and during the recruitment process, and that the consent you obtain is both voluntary and informed.

Recruiting colleagues as subjects

Work colleagues are best recruited on a face-to-face basis. In this regard it will be necessary for you to visit the research setting on all days of the week at times when day, evening and night staff will be available until you have recruited your sample. While this is both tiring and time consuming, it is by far the most informative and rewarding method of recruitment.

Like any recruitment exercise, when asking colleagues to participate, you should explain the purpose of the study and what will be required of them if they agree to take part. You must also reassure potential subjects that they may decline to participate, or withdraw from the study at any time without any fear of reprisal. During the recruitment interview, outline the provisions which will be made to guarantee the anonymity and confidentiality of the data, i.e. that the records will be kept secured and destroyed as soon as the statutory requirements for the storage of data have been met. As well, explain how the respondents will receive feedback about the outcome of the research.

When recruiting colleagues, it is wise to give them time to debate the pros and cons of participation amongst themselves before they make a commitment to your study. If you do this you should return to the research setting to answer any queries which may arise as a result of this debate before proceeding with the recruitment process.

Recruiting nurses not work colleagues

If your proposal calls for nurses as subjects, use frequently published hospital newsletters to bring your study to the notice of those who might meet the criteria for inclusion in the study population. While the practice of using subjects who are available and accessible (convenience sampling) is sometimes criticised as being open to bias, if you acknowledge this factor as a possible limitation to the generalisability of your findings, and use discretion in your advertising campaign, the problem can be minimised.

In order to avoid acquiring a biased sample, your advertisement should provide only broad guidelines as to who is required, e.g. 'the study has been designed to investigate the health profile of nurses' rather than 'the study has been designed to measure the incidence of back pain in nurses.' The latter approach may encourage nurses with back pain to volunteer! In your advertisement, inform the readers that more information is obtainable on request and, if contact is made, make all the details of the study available to the volunteer so as to allow them to give you their *informed* consent.

Recruiting patients as subjects

Preparation. Before approaching any patient for the purposes of recruitment, you should finalise two important tasks. If you have not already had to do so for IEC approval, prepare an information sheet which explains the purpose of the research, and what will be required of those participating in the study. In essence the contents of the sheet should echo what you plan to say during your recruitment session. You should therefore use terms a lay person can understand and include your contact telephone number or address, in case there are any problems or queries.

The second obligatory task is to inform the staff in the research setting of your proposed project. Your talk to staff should describe in detail any change of routine that will occur when the study is implemented. It should also provide enough information for them to answer questions about the study in your absence. During your talk, reinforce the fact that patients can withdraw at any time, and indicate whether the study is being undertaken by the agency for its own purpose, or by you for academic reasons and/or personal gain. After speaking with the staff, leave a copy of your approved proposal on the ward for their information and reference.

It is only when all ward staff have been given the opportunity to become acquainted with the project, and the majority can recognise you by sight, that you should begin recruiting your sample.

Approaching patients. Before you approach a patient for consent you should familiarise yourself with the literature regarding the patient's rights in research. These rights, described in many research text books, (e.g. Wilson's *Research in Nursing* 1989) were designed to protect patients from unethical research practices and encompass:

* the right to be informed;
* the right to full disclosure;
* the right to privacy, anonymity and confidentiality; and
* the right to self determination.

During the conduct of your study, the rights of patients must be upheld *at all times*. As such you should become familiar with the criteria attached to each of these rights and bear them in mind when approaching patients for consent.

When organising recruitment sessions, plan to visit each patient twice. During your initial contact, describe exactly what will be expected of those recruited for the study. Make it clear that participation in the study is not part of the patient's treatment. On no account should you exaggerate or

understate the risks, benefits, or requirements for participation. If you
can sense that a person is becoming
stressed as you outline the conditions, or is somewhat tentative about
committing him or herself after you
have explained the requirements, suggest that she or he does not take part
on this occasion. This strategy is a
useful one. It gives the person a reason
not to be a subject without having to
be the one to opt out. While this may
be a blow for your numbers, ethically
it is preferable, as you eliminate the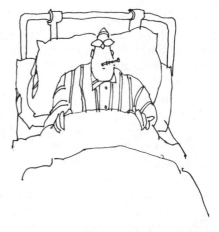
possibility of a subject feeling obligated to participate in the study.

Once you have described the conditions of participation, offer the patient
the option of either signing the consent form immediately, or taking more
time to think about participating in the study. If the patient wishes to delay
making a decision, leave the information sheet and the consent form with
him or her to be read at leisure and arrange a mutually convenient time to
return to collect the form, either signed or unsigned.

When it comes to signing the consent form, request that two copies be
signed. Leave the second copy with the patient for future reference.
Emphasise the fact that it is the patient's right to withdraw from the study
at any time *without penalty*. Make it easy to do this, by arranging for subjects
to tell any staff member that they no longer wish to participate. In the case
of outpatients, provide them with a telephone number where a message can
be left at any time.

When approaching new parents in the maternity setting, the use of an
additional strategy is sometimes useful. As new parents are extremely
protective of their babies, they are often very wary about allowing them to
become research subjects. Therefore, if your study requires neonatal
subjects, you may find it to your advantage to collect data from babies (for
whom you already have consent) where you can be seen by parents of
potential subjects, before you approach them for permission to collect data
from their infant.

Seeking informed consent in stressful circumstances, e.g. the labour ward
or immediately prior to surgery, is not recommended, unless it cannot be
avoided. Similarly, do not attempt to obtain consent from patients who have
been premedicated or sedated, or who are receiving other drugs which may
influence their ability to make an informed decision about participation.

If you have a choice, approach patients at a time when they can give you
their undivided attention, e.g. while waiting in the antenatal clinic or on the
day before surgery. If you do recruit patients away from the research setting,
however, you must remember that, although it may be a less stressful time,

your subjects may find it difficult to visualise the relevance and requirements of the study when they are remote from the reality of the situation. You will therefore need to explain all aspects of the project very carefully at the time of recruitment, and reiterate these when the patient qualifies for entry as a subject in your study.

On some occasions you may need to approach patients who may not ultimately be eligible for inclusion in the study. For example, if your sample requires individuals who have a malignancy, eligibility for entry to the study may not be confirmed until after a biopsy or similar diagnostic procedure. In these cases, if you elect to recruit subjects pre-operatively, you will need to approach all patients scheduled for these types of investigations, and confirm the patient's eligibility once the pathology results are known.

It is also important to recognise that wearing a nurse's uniform during recruitment interviews may influence the decision of a patient to participate. If patients incorrectly assume that a nurse's uniform automatically confers competency on the researcher to collect the required data, you may be open to the accusation of obtaining consent using an unfair advantage. Similarly if your uniform is perceived by patients as giving you the authority to influence their care, they may agree to participate, in fear that they may be disadvantaged in the future if they decline your offer.

Conversely, if you wear mufti, patients may not associate you directly with their care, or they may doubt your ability to perform the procedure/s for which your are seeking consent. Whether you elect to wear a uniform during recruitment is usually your decision. It may come down to whether you are working as a nurse at the time when you conduct the research. Whatever you decide it is *essential* that you always introduce yourself by name and status when you approach potential subjects, and advise them where you fit into the research setting.

Withholding information. Sometimes it is necessary to withhold precise information about a study to avoid bias in the results. For example, in a recent study conducted to determine whether the use of ice packs on puncture sites post cardiac catheterisation reduced discomfort, it was inappropriate to ask the patients who received ice packs following the procedure whether they had less discomfort than the group who were not given ice packs. In this study a non-committal approach to recruitment was used, viz:

> We want to try a new nursing procedure but I cannot tell you what it is. You may or may not get this new procedure in addition to the current, standard treatment. If you agree to participate I will visit you after data collection has been completed and tell you whether you received the new procedure.

By using this technique, patients had the right to refuse on the basis of a lack of information about the new procedure—a perfectly legitimate and acceptable reason not to participate. Inherent in the explanation, however, was an assurance that all standard treatment would be given regardless of whether the new procedure was used.

If you do need to withhold information about the nature of the procedure, remember that, unless patients are not in a position to compare notes about their treatment, you will need to ensure that all subjects in contact with each other (visual or other) receive the same treatment on the same day. If this is not possible, you may need to limit your recruitment of subjects to those who are isolated from others receiving the same treatment. This factor will considerably prolong your recruitment time, and you may choose to recruit all available subjects and allow for the information exchange element in the interpretation of your findings.

Recruiting children as subjects. Traditionally, parental consent alone has been sufficient for a child to become a study subject, but with the increasing recognition of the rights of children, parental consent alone is no longer necessarily considered to be sufficient. In her paper, Patricia Thompson (1987) provides guidelines for obtaining consent from children, based on their ability (competence) to make informed decisions about participating in research projects. These guidelines encompass:

- the anticipated benefit of the research for the subject;
- the degree of risk involved; and
- the likelihood that the child's privacy will be jeopardised during the collection of data.

In cases where the child may be expected to receive some benefit from the research (e.g. therapeutic studies such as drug trials), Thompson suggests that the person giving consent for participation will vary according to the competence of the child to make a decision and the risks/benefits involved in the study. Where the research is conducted to gain new knowledge without necessarily benefiting the patient subject (non-therapeutic research), Thompson acknowledges that, although children over the age of seven are generally competent enough to decide whether to participate, unless the child's privacy is an issue, the consent of both parent and child is necessary before the child can be included as a subject in the study.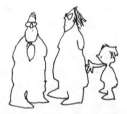

In most respects the methods used to recruit children for non-therapeutic research projects are similar to those used to recruit adults. If parental consent is required as well as that of the child, it is recommended that you obtain this (out of the child's hearing) prior to approaching the potential subject. This avoids disappointment should a parent refuse permission for participation.

When approaching a child for consent try and gain his or her confidence through informal, non-research-directed small talk before broaching the subject of participation. When you have established some rapport, present the information about the purpose of the study and the requirements for participation. Always use language appropriate to the child's developmental age. In the beginning this may take some practice—as some of the words used in the process of recruitment are not easy to explain (e.g. research).

As you would for adults, reassure children that their privacy and confidentiality will always be protected, and that their names will never be used when reporting the results of the study. You should also explain that there is no penalty if they choose not to participate and also that they may withdraw from the study at any time.

Be aware that some children may agree to participate merely to please you, or their parents who may be sitting by the bed. It is also important to remember that a child's refusal to participate in non-therapeutic research is usually considered to be absolute. Children compelled to participate in research studies sometimes jeopardise the validity of the data if they fail to complete the tasks to the best of their ability or, in the case of older children, sabotage the data they provide.

Recruiting subjects who are mentally impaired. As with children, undertaking research in the psychiatric setting brings with it extra challenges. Before committing yourself to recruiting subjects in the psychiatric setting, consider whether research can be carried out on an alternative study population. Where there is no alternative population, you will need to consider the criteria for inclusion in the study carefully, and define them clearly in your protocol. In determining these criteria, remember that patients who are manic, delusional, introverted or violent will not be capable of giving you informed consent. *Under no circumstances* should these patients be approached to participate in your study while they are manifesting any of these signs.

If you are interested in undertaking research on these patients during the acute phase of their condition, observation is the recommended method of data collection. Because observation is undertaken without the patients' consent, protocols using this method usually come in for close scrutiny by IECs before approval to conduct the study is granted. In this regard it will be up to you to convince the committee that the problem is significant, and that the benefits of the study will outweigh the fact that informed consent cannot be obtained from the patients.

Once the acute phase of their illness has passed however, many psychiatric patients are capable of understanding the purpose and requirements of your study. If this is the case, these patients may be recruited in the usual manner using appropriately worded consent forms which cater for the individual needs of prospective subjects.

Where a patient is suffering from a condition which is chronic and unlikely to improve enough for them to ever be able to give informed consent, you will need to enlist the co-operation of a next of kin or guardian. Try to ascertain the times when relatives are likely to be visiting the patient and return during this time to obtain their written consent. If this is not possible, contact the person responsible for the patient's welfare to explain the purpose of the study. If they agree to allow their relative to participate, request a meeting to sign the consent form.

Recruiting elderly subjects. If your research requires elderly persons to act as subjects, you will need to consider the factors associated with the ageing process which may influence the validity of your data, when formulating your inclusion criteria and recruitment strategies (Browning et al 1992). The decreased life expectancy of the elderly should also be considered, as this is likely to impact upon the retention rate of subjects recruited for longitudinal studies.

You should also keep in mind that a sample of institutionalised elderly subjects will generally return results which differ significantly from those provided by a sample drawn from the elderly population at large.

When determining your inclusion criteria, remember that in one elderly subject, there may be multiple pathologies present which may influence that individual's physiological or cognitive response to the 'dependant variable' (in the case of clinical trials) or the data collection instrument/s used in descriptive studies. Not surprisingly, confounding variables associated with disease processes are commonly encountered in elderly subjects who occupy acute hospital beds. Therefore if you choose to conduct research in this kind of setting, expect to be faced with the dilemma of having to separate the influences of chronological age and disease processes when working with elderly subjects.

Where, in spite of apparent drawbacks, the acute health care agency is still the most appropriate setting for your research, implement a pilot study to determine how the confounding variables will affect the quality of the data. If you choose to pursue a study which requires elderly subjects who have problems related to some specific medical condition, you really have no alternative but to collect the data and acknowledge any confounding variables as a limitation of your study.

On the other hand, if participation in the study does not depend on the presence of any specific pathology or other infirmity, avoid the health care settings which care for the acutely ill. Instead approach alternative agencies, (e.g. elderly citizens centres) which cater for the well elderly to obtain your sample.

Even in the absence of disease, increasing age requires that special consideration be given to individuals who meet your inclusion criteria. When preparing your information sheets and consent forms for use with elderly patients who are 'competent' enough to make an informed decision on their own behalf, print them in a slightly larger font (e.g. 15 point) than normal to enable those subjects with diminishing vision to read them. During the recruitment interview, you may also find that you will need to sit so as to maintain eye contact with the subject, and speak in a slightly louder voice than normal. By implementing these simple measures in addition to the normal recruitment strategies discussed earlier in this chapter, there is usually no problem in obtaining consent from a competent elderly patient when no one who can act as the person's advocate is present.

If the aging process has diminished the individual's intellectual capacity however, you will need to seek the co-operation of the patient's relative (or other person authorised to make decisions on their behalf) to ensure the patient's rights are, and are seen to have been, protected during the recruitment phase. The need to approach relatives for consent will depend on the potential subject's ability to give informed consent and to provide the required data. If you are unsure as to the status of the patient, check with the staff who are directly responsible for his or her care. Be guided by their assessment and advice, and if there is any question about the patient's competence, err on the safe side and enlist the assistance of the patient's relatives.

Relatives approached for consent should be provided with the same verbal and written information as competent patients. As in all recruitment exercises, it is essential that you establish some rapport with relatives before asking them to sign the consent form. This may be established either through informal conversation (possibly over a period of several days) or incidentally, as family members observe you collecting data from other patients without causing them harm or discomfort.

Due to a variety of moral, ethical and/or personal reasons, you may find some resistance by family members when asking them for permission to include their elderly relatives in your study. Often this is because of a fear that participation may incur unforeseen suffering during the collection of data. This situation has obvious implications for recruitment, but none that cannot be overcome by applying those recruitment strategies advocated earlier in this chapter, (e.g. timing, privacy, disclosure of information, etc.) when approaching the patient's relatives.

Extra subjects. On some occasions it may be tactful to approach individuals who do not meet your criteria for inclusion in the study. While this is not recommended if lengthy interviews are required, the administration of a short questionnaire or other data collection tool will often enable a person, not eligible for inclusion but eager to participate, to preserve their self esteem in a place where everyone else has been recruited for the study. This strategy is normally reserved for children. Being overlooked by a visitor who talks to every child in the room except them, is often a cause of acute disappointment for those ineligible to participate. If you do approach extra subjects for information however, be sure to flag the data they provide and consider it separately or remove it when processing your results.

Allocating your subjects to study groups

If your research involves the allocation of subjects to different study groups, the maintenance of equal group numbers is necessary to enable valid comparisons to be made between them.

Random numbers. Random numbers are commonly used to allocate subjects to groups. Lists of these numbers are readily available in research or statistics text books. In the interests of maintaining equal group numbers when the number of subjects required is only small, if you find three odd or three even numbers listed in a row, it is acceptable to go to next group of random numbers and recommence allocating your subjects using the alternative list.

Envelopes containing slips of paper which specify the name of the group to which the subject should be allocated are also commonly used in experimental studies. Providing the staff in the research setting are familiar with, and are prepared to co-operate in the allocation process, this method is a useful way of keeping groups equal. This is because should you lose a subject during the recruitment phase, you can add another envelope to the pile which contains the name of the group to which the former subject belonged. This strategy is reserved for instances where there is no obvious cause for the loss of subjects. Should an obvious reason appear, (e.g. withdrawal due to an adverse reaction to an experimental intervention) the future of the study should be considered—in the light of the factors contributing to the loss of subjects. Instruction in the allocation of subjects to their study groups in the pre-implementation education program is an essential part to the success of this method, as is a readily available supply of envelopes.

Medical record numbers. If you are working in a hospital setting, medical record numbers may also provide a basis for randomisation. If you plan to use identification numbers however, check to confirm their composition and method of allocation to patients before you implement your study. All the digits in the medical record number are not usually randomly allocated. In large networks where many agencies share the same patient identification system, some of the digits are commonly used to indicate the agency where an individual entered the system. To use this system successfully therefore, you must be aware of the composition of the number. With this information you will be able to avoid using those digits which are not randomly allocated and therefore eliminate the possibility of introducing a bias into the sample.

Matching subjects. If your study calls for nurses who select themselves for exposure to an intervention, you will need to match the nurses who volunteer themselves for the intervention (e.g. a special education program) with nurses who volunteer to participate in the study, but not to experience the intervention. Using relevant variables such as age, education, experience, designation and/or work area, you should build up a profile of each nurse and match those who will experience the intervention with those who will not. Allow for the possibility that members of the control group may drop out by matching two controls for every nurse in the experimental group. You should also select more potential control group members than you require, so that if members of this group drop out, there will still be sufficient numbers left to match your subjects for data analysis.

Implementing clinical research

Of all the different kinds of nursing research, the clinical trial offers the toughest challenge but some of the greatest rewards. Because the preparation phase is vital to the successful implementation of any clinically based study, it is outlined here in detail.

Preparing nursing staff

Ideally the study being implemented will have arisen from a problem in the research setting and the staff will have been involved in the planning phase. If you are external to the study setting, however, this may not be the case.

The more time you can spend with staff, explaining your research and the reasons for undertaking it, the smoother will be the implementation process.

Before implementing the study, it is essential that all permanent staff working in the research setting understand the purpose of your study, and the requirements of the data collection process associated with it. To ensure that everyone is familiar with the research methodology, you will need to visit the ward on all shifts on weekends and weekdays. The handover period is usually the most convenient time to speak to the staff but sometimes this is not possible. In these instances you will need to discuss your study with each nurse on an individual basis. Because you will not always be able to speak with casual staff, you should leave a copy of your proposal and any consent forms associated with it in a prominent place on the ward for reference. It may also be to your advantage to design a self learning package, containing the proposal and detailed information which fully explains the recruitment and data collection process, and leave it in the research setting for the staff to read at their leisure and refer to as the need arises.

During the familiarisation phase, try to emphasise the value of the research to the future practice of the nurses participating in the study. Where you can link the research problem directly to the nursing care delivered on the ward, (e.g. shorter time for procedures, reduced cost, increased patient comfort or reduced morbidity) your chances of co-operation will be enhanced. If during orientation however, you are unable to demonstrate any such link, it is likely that you have selected an inappropriate setting and consequently the chances of gaining the co-operation of the staff for data collection purposes will be extremely remote.

Calibration of equipment

If your study involves the use of equipment used for observations, e.g. thermometers, sphygmomanometers, watches, etc., you should test all the instruments likely to be used for data collection before you start, to determine any variations in the measurements they yield.

Follow the manufacturer's instructions exactly when testing the instruments. By doing this you will be more likely to detect the differences which occur between the different brand names. While many clinical measuring devices do vary, you should be comforted by the fact that the reliability of the data will be unaffected in studies requiring the detection of a change *within* individual patients. This is providing the same instrument is always used for the same subject, and all staff use the instrument as instructed.

For studies where the detection of a difference *between* patients is required, the extent to which the instruments vary becomes of greater importance. If after testing the equipment, you find that measurements are different enough to be clinically significant, select the most reliable instruments and clearly mark them so that the staff will know which equipment is being used for data collection purposes in your absence. Alternatively, you (and your biostatistician) can determine an acceptable confidence level for the observations and acknowledge the variation in measurements as a limitation of the study.

Ongoing management of clinical research

While you might want the nurses to own the research problem being studied, this does not mean that you can simply leave them to get on with collecting your data. Following the implementation of the study, you should maintain a high profile in the research setting, so that you can check that any required changes in practice are being adhered to, and sort out any early problems which may arise.

It is absolutely essential to its success that you continue to show your enthusiasm for your study throughout the *entire* data collection phase. In this regard try not to leave precious data lying around the ward for more than a day, and *never* for more than a week. By collecting data on a daily basis you raise your profile in the research setting and are readily available to answer questions about the conduct of the study. As a regular visitor, you can also become familiar with the work environment and any factors which may be limiting the collection of data. It is also good practice to give regular feedback about the progress of the study, either during the handover period or on a one-to-one basis, so that staff contributing data can see their efforts are not in vain. When it is deserved, give positive feedback to the staff. Filling up the ward lolly jar is one way of showing your appreciation for a job well done—as a reward for effort rather than as a bribe. Do not give rewards unless you are completely satisfied with the progress of the study. You may find that both the quantity and quality of the data falls off if the staff perceive a 'near enough is good enough' message in your rewards.

Providing your study is far enough advanced to show a definite trend, and if a suitable opportunity arises, another strategy for maintaining staff interest is to publish your interim results informally. A letter to the editor of a journal disseminating articles on a topic related to your research is a very practical way to acknowledge the contribution of the staff in an informal way. Where staff can see you value their efforts enough to publicise it, it is likely that they will be motivated to continue to provide data.

Collecting data by interview

If interviews are to be used to collect the data, you should consider whether highly specialised interview skills will be required to gather the required information. If this is the case, it may be worth your while to use trained interviewers. Although expensive, external interviewers have special skills in obtaining information and are not subject to any of the pressures exerted by the agency's hierarchy. In addition, subjects may be more willing to disclose information to someone without any prior knowledge of the organisation or its staff (providing they trust the interviewer to preserve confidentiality). If you choose to use outside interviewers however, you should plan to cross check every 10–20th interview with your data collector/s—to confirm that no bias is being inadvertently introduced during questioning.

Once you have obtained IEC approval, negotiate with your contact person in the research setting/s for a small space close to your population sample, where privacy, peace and quiet can be guaranteed during the conduct of the interviews. This is particularly important if you, or your interviewers, have no office in the research setting where privacy can be assured. In these circumstances subjects may be exposed to distraction, interruption or loss of privacy if interviews are conducted in a noisy, crowded outpatient department, or busy ward.

Setting up appointments

The key to obtaining useful data by interview is timing. Prior to conducting the interview, always negotiate an appointment time with your patients/clients which takes into account their physical condition, and the demands upon their time by other departments or appointments. When setting a time, remember that surgical patients in particular often tire very easily following a major procedure and/or a prolonged anaesthetic. These patients may not be able to complete interviews undertaken in the early post-operative period. In these cases, you should delay your meeting until the patient is well enough to tolerate questioning, and then keep your interview short and to the point.

Generally speaking, appointments during visiting hours are not recommended. The interview may be stifled or interrupted by the presence of family and friends, e.g. when new parents want to show off their babies, or otherwise enjoy the attention being lavished upon them. You may also find that, where a subject craves a rest rather than an interview, data obtained immediately after lunch may be less than satisfactory.

Bearing these limitations in mind, allow the subject to choose a mutually acceptable time to meet. Initially, contract with the person for one session only, and specify the length of time you expect the interview to take, so that you can leave politely if a lonely or talkative subject seeks to detain you.

Interviewing patients

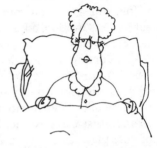

It is important to the success of the interview that you arrive on time and that your equipment is in good working order. If you are delayed, advise the subject as quickly as possible, so that they will be neither inconvenienced nor disgruntled by your failure to appear at the arranged time. If you plan to tape the interview, ensure you have enough tapes, and some spare batteries before you start.

Ensure privacy. Ideally interviews will be conducted in the private setting negotiated with your liaison person. It should be comfortable and without distractions, e.g. no telephone. Water should be available for refreshment. If you normally carry a page, you should turn it off, or arrange for someone to take your calls. The more distractions you can eliminate the better.

Ensure confidentiality. Just as nurses will need to trust the credibility of the researcher before divulging sensitive information, patients will need to develop a similar level of trust before revealing personal details. You should therefore reinforce the arrangements which will ensure the confidentiality of their information before beginning your interview.

Taping an interview. Consent to tape an interview must be obtained during the recruitment phase. After you have re-established rapport, and the interview begins to warm up, turn on the tape recorder and remind your subject of the purpose of the interview, and of the presence of the tape recorder. This introductory phase is useful as it confirms the consent to record in a different form. It also allows subjects to become used to the recorder, to such an extent that they may soon forget about its presence.

Obtaining consent to record an interview session does not necessarily mean the subject is comfortable with the arrangement. When discussing personal or otherwise sensitive issues, you may find it to your advantage to turn the recorder off and take notes by hand. Negative body language, hesitancy of speech, or vague responses, not qualified after supplementary questioning, may all be signs of a need to discontinue taping the interview.

Interviewing subjects at home. In certain circumstances you may need to visit a subject at home to collect your data. If this becomes necessary, avoid making an appointment around meal times, very early in the morning—when some people are still collecting their thoughts, or late in the day, when you may find people pushed for time or tired from work. If you choose to make an appointment during the weekend, you should remember that this is often a busy time for families, and consequently you may find yourself with only a limited time to conduct the interview. Whatever the time however, it is in your interest to confirm the appointment before you set out on your visit. It may save you a fruitless journey if your subject has overlooked the agreed time, or for some reason, changed his or her mind.

Conducting an interview at home has advantages for both the subject who is more likely to feel relaxed in familiar territory, and the interviewer who has the opportunity to gain insight into the subject's ecology. It is a privilege to be invited into a private home, and as such you should aim to be as unobtrusive as possible. In busy households, you will need to find a quiet private place (the garden can be ideal in fine weather), as you may find yourself interviewing more than one member of the family.

Occasionally it may be necessary to find some neutral ground to conduct your interview. If the subject's home or your research setting is inconvenient, the local park or a convenient coffee shop will suffice, providing privacy and comfort can be maintained during the interview.

Interviewing nurses in the work setting

If you have permission to interview nurses during work time, allow them to choose their interview times, and always be prepared for a change of time at short notice. When visiting the ward to arrange an appointment or conduct an interview, be aware that an unexpectedly heavy work load may preclude any meaningful contact with the nursing staff. If this situation does arise, write your telephone or page number on a slip of paper and give it to your subject, inviting him or her to contact you at a more convenient time. Do not insist on keeping your appointment as your 'victim' may agree to talk to you only to get rid of you, with the result that both the data and any chance of future co-operation will invariably suffer. Never visit a work area without warning and expect nurses to be available for interview. Where you respect their need to do their job, it is likely that nurses will do their best to co-operate with you.

Subjects with special needs

Collecting data from children

When designing a data collection instrument for use with children, it is not enough to have a good knowledge of research methodology. It is vital to the success of your study that the construction and administration of the data collection instruments take into account the unsophisticated and immature nature of children and incorporate the theories of child development put forward by psychologists such as Piaget, Erikson and Mahler. This is because the validity of the data collected will almost certainly be jeopardised if the demands of research tasks exceed the child's developmental capabilities.

Working with toddlers. When devising proposals which use toddlers as subjects, remember that the chances of co-operation using standardised tools are minimal. This is because toddlers:

- assume everyone's outlook is exactly the same as their own;
- have only a short attention and memory span;
- cannot deal with abstract thoughts;
- process information using representational thought, i.e. all dogs resemble their dog, all tricycles resemble their tricycle etc.; and
- are concerned only with the here and now and have no concept of time, space or sequence.

The data collection method which best acknowledges these limitations is naturalistic observation—behind one way mirrors. Observational methods (usually of play) have the potential to yield information on various aspects of behaviour such as communication, skill attainment or activities. Although it can be argued there are ethical issues involving consent when collecting data from children using observation, the method is favoured for its ability to yield valid data in difficult circumstances, providing the observations are not subject to bias or distortion.

Modifying standardised tools for use by children

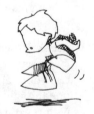

With increasing age, it becomes more feasible to use standardised methods of data collection—provided these are modified to accommodate the developmental characteristics of the age group being studied. Until the age of approximately seven years, children do not understand the factors of consistency and reliability, and therefore tend to want to undertake tests their way rather than conform to a set of prescribed instructions, e.g. sitting on a lap rather than at a table. This limitation has implications for the research design in that it demands that you should standardise the responses to your data collection instrument—rather than attempt to standardise the conditions under which data is collected.

Because young children tend to score high on liar detection tests, avoid incorporating social desirability scales in your data collection instrument. If you choose to use these scales, it is likely the results you obtain will only represent what the child thinks will please you, rather than the actual truth.

Aspects of test administration

When approaching a child for consent, or to collect data, try to gain some rapport with him or her at your earliest opportunity. While small talk or appropriate toys, books or games may help you break the ice, remember that non-verbal cues will be equally important in establishing a good relationship with your subject. From your earliest contact, it is extremely important to gain the trust of the child—especially if more than one contact is envisaged. Remember that the growth of this trust will be facilitated if the explanation of the required task ultimately measures up to the child's expectation. Where the researcher has gained the trust of the child, co-operation is more likely, and valid data will be the reward during subsequent interactions. On the other hand, if the task does not live up to expectations, it is likely that the co-operation you may have enjoyed during the initial contact will disappear.

As with adults, timing is important when collecting data from children. The attention span of young children is only five to seven minutes and may be influenced by tiredness and hunger. You must therefore avoid the potential for these factors to influence your data collection. Mid morning is an ideal time for testing, when children are normally alert and active. Try to avoid testing subjects immediately after lunch or during the traditional rest period in hospital, as the child may be sleepy or otherwise in need of a rest.

Other factors to consider when collecting data from children are that visual stimuli will provide a major distraction for the young child, as will a full bladder. Therefore, wherever possible, collect your data in a setting which is familiar to the child (e.g. the ward rather than your office). Ensure too that a visit to the toilet is not required or precedes the testing process.

When giving directions during data collection *always*:

- use vocabulary appropriate to the child's developmental age;
- use short sentences and concrete language;
- avoid sentences which contain double negatives and exceptions;
- test your variables sequentially. Children are capable of processing only one thought at a time, therefore tests which ask young children to deal with several tasks simultaneously are likely to result in poor quality data;
- supplement explanations with illustrated materials or demonstrations whenever possible—as children react better to visual rather than verbal cues.

Even when using these guidelines, you should always keep in mind that the answer provided may not necessarily be the answer to the question you asked—but rather the children's interpretation of it. Consequently you may receive some surprising responses, which will require you to reword your question/s so as to achieve a more uniform interpretation of their content by the study subjects.

As mentioned previously, most young children are keen to please and will respond well to positive reinforcement. You should therefore be prepared to offer small rewards such as stickers, certificates, pencils or balloons for appropriate efforts, e.g. for concluding a test, reaching a standard or as motivation (not a bribe) to continue providing data.

Collecting data from elderly subjects

When designing a data collection instrument for use with elderly subjects, it is essential that the instrument/s used to collect the data take into account any factors associated with ageing that are likely to influence the validity of the data. As in the case of children, if the demands of research tasks exceed the subject's capabilities, the quality of the data will almost certainly be compromised.

Modifying standard tools for use by the elderly

When devising proposals which require elderly subjects, you should remember that, although members of your study population may meet the physical criteria for inclusion, within this potential sample there will be a wide range of reading, comprehension and/or other cognitive skills. Until recently it was commonly believed that data collection tools for use with the elderly should be designed for use by those subjects with the least cognitive ability. Phillips (1992) however has reported that this strategy is not as useful as it was once thought because:

- if data collection instruments are excessively tailored to cater for a very small number of subjects, the modified instruments can incur a loss of face validity for the majority of subjects, who have normal reading and comprehension skills;
- the oversimplification of responses has been known to confuse competent subjects who find themselves unable to complete simple tasks because of a lack of alternatives or opportunity to provide the appropriate response;
- in studies where researchers reported difficulties obtaining data from the elderly using more complex instruments, e.g. semantic differential or Likert (type) scales, the problems could often be attributed to the manner in which the tasks or questions were presented to the subject.

In particular, differences between the frames of reference of the investigator and the subject are identified by Phillips (1992) as commonly contributing to the failure of subjects to provide the required data. Furthermore, questions presented out of context, or ones which are irrelevant to the subject, have been reported as being particularly troublesome to many elderly subjects.

The implications of these observations are that any data collection instrument designed for use with the elderly should be as simple as it needs to be to obtain valid data from the *majority* of respondents. Furthermore the content should be relevant to the subject's sphere of existence, and placed within a familiar context, to avoid the possibility of confusing or overwhelming those individuals providing the data. To achieve these standards, more than one pilot study may be necessary before you have enough information to construct an instrument which has the potential to return valid data. In this regard, at least one pilot study and a validation exercise are *essential* if your tool is to be used successfully during your study.

Format of data collection instruments for use by the elderly. If your work with elderly subjects involves questionnaires or other written information, you should ensure that the size of the print is large enough to be read by those subjects who are visually impaired. While any questionnaire should be printed in at least a 12 point font, those designed for use with the elderly should be at least 15 points.

example   12 point font

15 point font

Aspects of test administration

When collecting data from elderly subjects, allow enough time to chat with the person before attempting to distribute a questionnaire or commence an interview. Most institutionalised elderly will enjoy an opportunity to talk with a visitor, and you should use this period to gain rapport with your subject before beginning the collection of data. As is the case for children, your non-verbal cues will be as important as anything you say in gaining the trust of your subject. You should therefore remain aware of this fact during the warm up phase.

Where possible include the subject's relatives in the collection of data. Providing there is no potential for the validity of the data to be compromised, relatives can be a useful ally during this phase. At the same time they may be reassured of the innocuous nature of the tasks required by the research.

As with all subjects, timing is important when collecting data from the elderly. While you may find some of your subjects have only limited attention spans, others may tire easily. Be aware of the potential for these factors to influence your data and therefore, where possible, avoid testing subjects during visiting hours, immediately after lunch or during the traditional rest period in hospital.

Another factor to consider when collecting data from elderly subjects is that of privacy. A loss of hearing will sometimes cause a person to raise their voice above the usual volume. For this reason you should seek to conduct your interview out of the ward setting—in your designated space. Otherwise the potential may exist for a breach of confidentiality or an invasion of other people's privacy.

Optimising data collection using questionnaires

In Chapter 7, the development of questionnaires is discussed in detail. In addition to the content and format of the instrument however, there are certain organisational and administrative aspects of questionnaire design which should also be considered before you implement your study.

Instructions to respondents

As survey participants generally appreciate a uniform method of response, if possible try to keep method of answering similar throughout the question-naire. If this is not possible, clear instructions for answering each question should be included each time the method of response changes, for example:

Q1.   What is your age in years?
       (Fill in the box provided)

Where terms are open to interpretation (e.g. senior, regular, severe), include a definition for each term with the question, for example:

Q2.   What is your current position? (Circle one number)
       Clinical Nurse Specialist   1
       Clinical Nurse   2
       * Senior Registered Nurse   3
       +Junior Registered Nurse   4
       Enrolled Nurse   5

       * Senior Registered Nurse:- more than 3 years nursing experience
       + Junior Registered Nurse:- less than or equal to 3 years nursing experience

If you are prepared to allow for more than one response in a question, make this clear in the instructions, for example:

Q3.   What cues do you use to assess a patient's pain?
       (Circle as many numbers as you wish)
       Patient's complaints of pain   1
       Patient's facial expression   2
       Patient's body position   3
       Patient's pulse rate   4
       Your own instinct   5
       Other (please specify)   6

If concepts are difficult to explain or unfamiliar to the respondents, e.g. the 10 cm long Visual Analogue Scale (VAS), give an example as a guide. Make sure that the example *clearly illustrates* your requirements, for example:

Q4.   Mark a cross on the line at the point which indicates the level of your pain right
       now.

       No pain   Worst pain
       at all   imaginable
       (This patient has indicated severe pain)

If not all questions need to be answered by every study subject, filter questions may be used to direct your respondents to only those questions which they need to answer. Filter questions have the advantage of elimi-nating the need for respondents to read questions which are irrelevant to them. They also serve to confirm any subsets within the population sample that may have been identified during the development of the proposal, for example:

Q5.   Do you work permanent night duty? (Circle one number)
       Yes   1   Go to Q6.
       No   2   Go to Q12 on page 4.

A 'yes' response immediately identifies the night duty subset. In addition, those respondents who do not work permanent night duty are directed past questions 6–11 which relate only to that duty.

For questions which seek to measure a degree of intensity (none–worst); frequency (never–always); or preference (agree–disagree), an ordinal scale may be used to rank the subject's responses along a continuum.

The form and sensitivity of ordinal scales is dependant upon the attribute being measured. The VAS line depicted in Q4 is an example of a simple but, in the absence of designated 'scale steps' a highly sensitive measure. Anchored by the two opposite ends of the pain continuum, there are 100 possible responses to the 10 cm VAS line, as the response is measured in millimetres from the left anchor, 'No pain'.

Less sensitive but easier to analyse, are scales which incorporate 'scale steps' anchored by numbers for example:

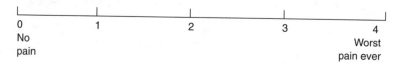

```
0              1              2              3              4
No                                                          Worst
pain                                                        pain ever
```

or by words (which can be coded as numbers for analysis):

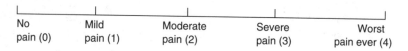

```
No             Mild           Moderate       Severe         Worst
pain (0)       pain (1)       pain (2)       pain (3)       pain ever (4)
```

Scales may also be anchored by degrees of agreement or disagreement, for example: *Strongly Agree, Agree, (Uncertain), Disagree, Strongly Disagree, (Don't Know)*; or by adverbs for example: *Always, Frequently, Sometimes, Never.*

In recent times, many different scales, each unique in their degree of complexity, sensitivity and sophistication, have been developed to measure a wide variety of social/psychological traits. If you choose to include a scale in your questionnaire, you should consult a research methodology text for more detailed information about their use. Always remember however that, as highly sensitive instruments tend to fragment the responses, this may give rise to problems during data analysis if the sample size is small. (See Ch. 7.)

Supplementary information

If you choose to recruit your subjects before distributing your questionnaire, the inclusion of a descriptive paragraph at the beginning of the question-naire which includes a brief overview of the study and a reminder of the agreement to participate in the study is usually sufficient to refresh your subject's memory. Where no previous contact with the subject has occurred however, you will need to enclosed a separate covering letter seeking the co-operation of the subject.

The covering letter. The letter which accompanies the questionnaire should be personally addressed to each individual selected to participate in the study. Its content should describe the background to the study, the problem being investigated and how the results will be used. If you have randomly chosen your sample, explain how subjects were selected to participate, i.e. which list was used to select the names, (roster, phone book, etc.) and give your reassurance that the data obtained will be kept confidential and that the results will be reported in such a way as to protect the identity of the participants. Make it clear where replies are to be sent or left, and include a deadline for the receipt of replies (which is a little earlier than when you really want them). Wherever possible sign the letter personally in blue ink (Dillman 1978). Your personal signature is an indication that the invitation to participate in the study comes from a human being rather than a photocopier and is therefore recommended.

If you are asking people to mail their completed questionnaires back to you, plan to include either a stamped self addressed, or a reply paid, envelope of suitable dimensions. Of these options, the latter offers the greatest advantage. Apart from a small service fee, you are required to pay postage only if the questionnaire is returned, thereby saving you the cost of supplying stamps that may never be used for their intended purpose.

Preparing a questionnaire for printing

Only when you have completed the pilot study, should you contemplate the mass production of your questionnaire and the letter which is to accompany it at the point of distribution. Printing can be a costly component of a research budget and therefore you will need to ensure that the copy that you give to the printer is valid, user friendly and as attractive as possible.

If you are preparing your questionnaire on a word processor and have access to a laser printer, it is likely you will have the choice of a wide range of typefaces and fonts. Making the correct choice is important, as some typefaces| are easier to read than others. In their comprehensive guide to typesetting, Grazier and Yelland (1993) offer useful advice regarding the production of documents by computer. As the information is relevant to the preparation of questionnaires, it is presented here for your consideration.

Typeface. Choose a simple typeface; e.g. Helvetica or Times, and use it consistently throughout the questionnaire. As a general rule it is not advisable to mix your typefaces, e.g. between the modest Courier and the flamboyant Futura, or even between the popular Times and Helvetica. The change in the appearance of the letters may be enough to distract your reader from the purpose of the question and detract from the quality of the data.

Use of capitals. Reserve the use of UPPER CASE for headings or emphasis. Apart from adding up to 35% to the space requirements, capitals are slower and more difficult to read when used for large blocks of text.

Size of the letters (point size). Choose a letter size which will suit the study population. As age increases so should the size of the letters—to about a 15-point size. Avoid making the letters so large that the questions consume excessive numbers of lines. In long questionnaires this will add substantially to the number of pages and therefore printing costs.

Emphasis of your chosen typeface. If you want to emphasise words or phrases, use the *italics version* . Do not overdo the emphasis however. Not only will it slow down reading time, but the thrust of the point may also be lost if you hide it in large blocks of text.

Length of the lines. If the lines are too short in blocks of text, the eyes cannot run over the words easily. Conversely long lines tire the eyes and make it difficult to concentrate on the task. 55–60 characters per line is recommended or, where large typeface is used, up to 2.5 times the point size.

Line spacing. While the use of space is recommended, use it sparingly, for example, around the actual questions. Widely spaced text may interrupt the flow as the eyes look for the next line. Conversely, if the text is too close, there is the risk of reading more than one line at a time.

Proof reading questionnaires

As well as conforming to the principles of good layout, your questionnaire should have face validity. Poor grammar and spelling mistakes can detract from the appeal of your questionnaire and you should therefore aim to eliminate both of these factors through meticulous proof reading before you submit your forms to the printer.

Providing you have established the appropriate form of validity for your questionnaire, friends who are not nurses usually make very good proof readers because they cannot read in the missing words or steps, to comprehend your questions. In addition to seeking feedback on the ease of use and appearance of the form, ask your proof reader to check for spelling mistakes. Do not merely rely on the word processor's spell check facility to detect spelling errors as words which are correctly spelled but out of syntax are normally not recognised by this process, e.g. signing/singing, tiger/timer, fur/fir. While singing the consent form may be an innovative recruitment strategy, IECs will normally expect subjects to sign it, so be sure to scrutinise each page carefully before sending it to the printer.

Printing questionnaires

Before visiting a printer, determine what colour/s, what size and what quality paper you require. You will also need to decide what format you want the questionnaire to take. (Where funds permit, a large questionnaire can be made to look smaller by having it printed in a booklet format.) If your study calls for the distribution of questionnaires to different groups, or the redistribution of the same questionnaire on more than one occasion, consider printing the forms in different colours. It will make the compilation and processing of the forms much easier.

Given that the quality of the paper you choose will enhance (or detract from) the face validity of your questionnaire, select the best quality bond you can afford. If you plan to print the questionnaire on both sides of the paper, you will require a heavy bond. Light weight paper tends to absorb the ink and therefore cannot be successfully 'backed'. Before committing yourself to a printer, shop around, as there can be a wide variation in the price of printing. Instant printing is sometimes expensive, and you may find it much cheaper to use a slower service. When getting quotes, be sure the price includes any collating, stapling, folding, etc. which may be required. It will also be to your advantage if there is good access to parking at the print shop, as questionnaires are extremely heavy to carry long distances.

When negotiating a price, remember that, as a printed form, question-naires incur sales tax. In this regard, if you are a member of staff at your research setting, it may pay you to investigate the possibility of having the supply department arrange your printing for you. In certain cases they may be able to claim a tax exemption on your behalf. Regardless of who organises the job, however, be sure to set a delivery deadline well before you actually plan to distribute the questionnaires, to offset any unexpected delays which may arise.

Strategies for matching questionnaires

If your study entails the repeated administration of a questionnaire to the same subjects, you will need to employ a coding system to enable the questionnaires to be matched for analysis at the conclusion of the survey. One strategy to achieve this end is to group the questionnaires into sets and code each set before distribution.

For example, if pre- and post-intervention surveys are required and 150 subjects are required to complete both questionnaires, have all the forms printed at the same time. Before distribution, code the questionnaires from 1–150 using 'a' and 'b' to denote whether the response is a pre- or post-test, i.e. 300 forms grouped into 150 sets numbered from 1a and 1b through to 150a and 150b. Alternatively you can have the forms printed in different colours to distinguish between each phase of the study. In this case sets will comprise two questionnaires, each of a different colour, but marked only with a number. (Colour coding will make the letter coding unnecessary.)

During the distribution phase, ask the subject to select a set of question-naires. Following this selection, provide an envelope large enough to hold the questionnaire and ask the person to address the envelope to him or herself. Place the second questionnaire (and a covering letter reminding the subject of their participation in the study) in the envelope, stick it down and retain it. When it is time to conduct the second phase of the study, simply mail all the pre-addressed envelopes and match the replies using the number codes as they are returned.

For studies which use nurses as subjects, obscure dates, known only to the respondents (e.g. mother's date of birth), may be requested for coding purposes. Alternatively subjects can be asked to choose their own form of identification symbol. Although this is by far the most entertaining form of coding for the researcher, it relies on the subjects remembering their personalised symbols between administrations of the questionnaires, and is therefore not so suitable for studies which extend over long periods. In all cases the second questionnaire should be accompanied by an explanatory letter, which reminds the participants about the original study. Never send follow up questionnaires *without* any explanatory information.

Distributing questionnaires to staff

When distributing questionnaires in hospitals and other health care agencies, it will be to your advantage to meet those staff members selected in your sample personally. This will enable you to directly sell your study to the staff, who will then have the advantage of being able to visualise the person asking the questions. If this is not possible, the covering letter which accompanies the questionnaire should be personally addressed to each selected staff member.

If you are external to the hospital or agency, arrange a time to visit the setting to distribute the forms. If possible, arrange for a staff member to accompany you into the work areas. It will give you credibility if the staff can identify with a familiar face who is, by their presence, seemingly supporting your research.

On D day (distribution day), start early and wear comfortable shoes, as the process will always take longer than you expect. If your questionnaires are individually addressed, group them by floor and ward or department and arrange the forms in the order that you will visit each area before you start. As questionnaires are usually heavy, do not try to carry all the forms at once as your arms will tire very quickly. Instead negotiate to leave the bulk of the forms in a safe place and make several short trips rather than one long one. In a multi story building, leave the forms on a middle level and work from the upper to the lower floors.

Maximising questionnaire distribution by staff

If the collection of your data is dependant on the distribution of a question-naire or similar document by staff, you will need to ensure that sufficient supplies of the forms are available in all study settings at all times. While being employed in the setting makes this relatively easy to achieve, if you are external to the organisation, it will be in your best interest to establish a contact person in each of the settings where the forms are being distributed. Once the study is implemented telephone your contact person, or visit the setting regularly to check that sufficient forms are available for distribution.

Arrange to have the forms (or a reminder to distribute them) kept within easy reach of the staff who are distributing them on your behalf. It is unreasonable to expect them to photocopy your questionnaires to replenish the supply, and to do so will result in a poor response rate. The onus is on you to ensure that questionnaires are always available for distribution during the data collection period.

Optimising return rates by patients

For studies where feedback from patients is required about aspects of performance, e.g. satisfaction surveys or competency studies, some members of your sample may fear reprisal from staff if they give negative feedback. In these cases, assume the responsibility for the distribution of the forms yourself. When explaining the study, emphasise the fact that the data will remain confidential to the researcher and the results will be reported so as to protect the identity of the participants. It should be said that respondents are often more willing to volunteer information to a person whom they see as having no influence upon their care. If you have no connection with the research setting—other than the conduct of your research, say so. It may reassure the subject that there will be no reprisals if their replies indicate an element of dissatisfaction about the care they are receiving.

Whatever method you choose to administer the questionnaire, demonstrate your commitment to the confidentiality of the data by providing a means for return which ensures privacy. Envelopes which can be sealed by respondents, sturdy boxes for the receipt of replies and a coding system which effectively conceals the subject's identity are all means which reinforce your message of confidentiality and subsequently contribute to an increase in the return rate.

Using commercial carriers

Generally it is in the best interests of research undertaken by the survey method to distribute questionnaires so that they reach all research subjects simultaneously. If you need to send questionnaires over long distances, make an appointment to see the manager of your chosen carrier service before you attempt to send questionnaires to rural and/or remote areas. Explain what the research is trying to achieve and the importance of the material arriving safely at its destination. You should also find out the estimated date of delivery so that you can coordinate the distribution to coincide with the arrival of the forms outside the metropolitan area. Where special service or favours are given, a thank you is always indicated.

Incentives

While financial incentives should not normally be offered to study subjects in return for their participation in your study, patients and/or staff often delight in small tokens of thanks for the data they provide. Tea bags, stickers, pencils, chocolate frogs or other small items are usually appreciated by study subjects and you should therefore consider a tangible way of repaying them for their time when implementing your data collection strategies.

Conclusion

In this chapter, we have discussed those factors which contribute to the success of clinical nursing research. Each aspect of the research process which has been found by experienced nurse researchers to facilitate the implementation and conduct of clinical studies has been discussed in some detail. As it is these factors which exert the greatest influence on the success of your study, it is essential that each be carefully addressed when implementing studies in the clinical area.

REFERENCES

Abdellah F, Levine E 1986 Better patient care through nursing research, 3rd edn. MacMillan, New York
Australia Post 1993 List of lists, 4th edn. Advertising mail Unit, Australia Post, Melburne
Browning C, Kendig H, Minichiello V 1992 Research methods in gerontology. In: Minichiello V, Alexander L, Jones D (eds) Gerontology: a multidisciplinary approach. Prentice Hall, New York
Dillman D 1978 Mail and telephone surveys: the total design method. John Wiley, New York
Educational Computing Services, Curtin University of Technology 1990 How to design a questionnaire for computer analysis. Curtin University of Technology, Perth WA
Field P, Morse J 1992 Nursing research: the application of qualitative approaches. Chapman and Hall, London
Grazier B, Yelland J 1993 Typo survival kit—for all TYPE emergencies. Press for Success, South Perth WA
Phillips L 1992 Challenge of nursing research with the elderly. Western Journal of Nursing Research 14(6):720–730
Thompson P 1987 Protection of the rights of children as subjects for research. Journal of Pediatric Nursing 2(6):392–399
Waltz C, Strickland O, Lenz R 1991 Measurement in nursing research, 2nd edn. F A Davis, Philadelphia
Wilson H 1989 Research in nursing, 2nd edn. Addison Wesley, Redwood City
Van Ort S 1981 Research design: pilot study. In: Krampitz S, Pavlovich M (eds) Readings for nursing research. Mosby, St Louis

6. Common problems in the clinical setting

Western Australian Nurse Researchers' Network

Regardless of its anticipated benefits for patient care, every aspect of research conducted in a clinical setting carries with it the potential to encounter problems and pitfalls. While minor difficulties may simply hinder your progress, those having a significant influence may ultimately cause your study to fail.

The recruitment of the study sample and the collection of data can be a source of much frustration and disappointment during the conduct of a clinical study. Most commonly researchers encounter problems related to the recruitment and retention of subjects, and with subjects and staff who do not comply with the requirements of the research. Problems within the research setting, however, may also disrupt the collection of data. These difficulties, coupled with the challenges associated with confronting subjects who are blatantly unco-operative, whose primary language is not English or who are particularly unwell can make the collection of data a particularly trying experience.

Anticipation of potential problems is the key to minimising the anxiety associated with the conduct of studies in the clinical area. This chapter addresses some of the problems researchers commonly face during the collection of data, and suggests strategies to facilitate this crucial aspect of the research process.

Recruitment and retention of subjects

Slow recruitment

Of all the problems that researchers face, the recruitment and retention of subjects provides the greatest number of headaches. As a general rule, the recruitment of your study sample will usually take longer than you anticipate. This is usually because either:

- persons who meet the criteria for inclusion in the population sample do not present themselves at the study setting; or
- staff in the research setting vested with recruitment responsibilities fail to approach subjects when and if they present at the setting.

Delays in finalising the collection of data which arise as a result of slow recruitment may not be a problem for those investigators conducting research in their own work setting. For students however, they can result in an extra financial burden if re-enrolment becomes necessary due to the failure to recruit the required sample size before the submission deadline is reached. By implementing a few simple strategies in the planning stage of the study, problems associated with recruitment can be minimised and the required sample obtained within the proposed time frame.

Insufficient potential subjects

Before deciding upon a research setting, it is essential that you ascertain the number of potential subjects who can be expected to attend the setting within the allocated time frame. As a general rule, unless the agency has the potential to provide at least twice the number of subjects required to fulfil the requirements for your sample size in the time available consider:

- approaching an alternative setting where sufficient subjects will be available for recruitment within the available time; or
- selecting a second, comparable setting where there will be sufficient additional subjects to supplement the numbers available at the original location.

While either of these options are acceptable, an alternative setting may not be available to you. In this case you will need to reconsider the significance of the problem you wish to investigate. If your reasons for undertaking the research are still valid then you will need to readjust the time frame for your research to accommodate the likelihood of slow recruitment.

When assessing the potential of a health care agency to provide the required number of subjects, you should also consider the impact your study might have on the use of the setting. For example, in a recent clinical trial which sought to evaluate various methods of treating lacerations, the recruitment rate slowed significantly as the clientele of the research setting became aware of the study and sought treatment in alternative agencies, rather than face being recruited for the study. While this scenario is the exception rather than the rule, it does indicate the potential of the local grapevine to influence your rate of recruitment in those areas serviced by a single health care agency and this factor should be taken into consideration when deciding on a setting.

Eligible subjects not approached

If sufficient numbers of the study population attend the setting but are not approached to participate in the study, your anticipated recruitment rate will also suffer. This problem is commonly encountered where the researcher is not employed in the research setting and is relying on the staff to recruit subjects on his or her behalf. In these cases the difficulties usually stem from the fact that, as the nurses do not own the problem being researched, they are less committed to the study than if it were their own. Where staff regard the research problem as being incidental to their practice, it is likely they will regard the recruitment of subjects as extra work which is extraneous to their usual role. As such the signing up of study subjects may be given a low priority in a busy clinical setting and recruitment rates may suffer as a result.

This problem is difficult to remedy once a study has been implemented and you should therefore choose a setting where staff value the reason for your research and are supportive of its aims. Usually it will work to your advantage if staff regard the question or hypothesis under scrutiny as being new, different or timely.

If you are planning to ask staff in the research setting to recruit patients on your behalf, you must be prepared to spend whatever time is necessary to convince them of the merits of your project. The success you have in selling them the benefits of the study will be ultimately reflected in their contribution to your project. If staff are ambivalent to your research and recruitment is slow because potential subjects are not being approached to participate, the onus will fall back on you to recruit your own subjects, distribute your own questionnaires, and perform any other tasks previously assigned to the staff. This extra effort is well worthwhile. Not only will you reach your required sample size faster, but you will also personally experience any problems associated with your data collection instrument, and will be better informed to deal with any difficulties should they arise. If you are called upon to recruit your own subjects, the strategies outlined in Chapter 5 should help you boost the rate of recruitment.

Retention of subjects

In longitudinal studies the depletion of subject numbers during the course of the research can cause major problems during data analysis. Ultimately the loss of subjects can jeopardise the outcome of the study. Therefore, if you need to see patients after discharge, check to see where they plan to be at the time of the follow up appointment *before* they are discharged. Never assume your subject will always return to his or her home to recuperate as this is not always the case.

If you do lose track of a subject, try contacting the person nominated as next of kin in the medical record to ascertain their whereabouts. If this person cannot help you, do not despair. They are not the only (or necessarily the best) source of information. There are often other avenues to pursue before you have to withdraw a lost subject from your study. The clues to a patient's whereabouts will vary, depending on the individual circumstances. Reading the medical record (with the appropriate permission) should provide you with additional ideas, such as the type of aftercare the subject was expected to receive and the agencies scheduled to provide it. Such information may enable you to locate the subject and complete your data collection.

During the course of a clinical study, if you find that subjects are withdrawing from the study, try to identify the reasons—particularly if those retiring are all from one group. Where possible eliminate the cause, but if this is not feasible, report how many subjects were lost, and the factors contributing to the loss, when you write up your findings.

Disruption of the research setting

Loss of setting

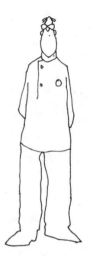

Even worse than the loss of subjects, is the loss of the research setting. It can have devastating if not lethal consequences for your study. There are many reasons why you might lose access to the setting. Some can be foreseen, e.g. ward renovation, whilst others are totally unexpected, e.g. flooding caused by a burst water main. To minimise this possibility, it is essential that, during your initial visit to the setting, you confirm that it will be available for at least the expected duration of your data collection.

If it is discovered during the planning stage of the study that access to the chosen setting will be temporary, or the loss of setting can be otherwise foreseen, either seek access to a second placement before you commence data collection, or find another setting which will be available to you for the duration of the study.

Should your source of subjects be cut off unexpectedly, you have three realistic alternatives. If you have nearly completed collecting data, you can stop the study and process the results you have to hand. This is only an option however, if the numbers of subjects are sufficient to give you meaningful results from which valid conclusions can be drawn.

For studies which are not so far advanced, relocation to an alternative setting is your only viable option. This is a lengthy process however, which will require you to seek out and assess new locations and obtain permission from the governing institutional ethics committees.

Before committing yourself to an alternative venue, ensure that the prevailing conditions are similar enough to the original setting to enable the data from both places to be combined. You must therefore be able to minimise or eliminate any confounding variables which exist in either setting, to enable this to occur.

In cases where you are able to find an alternative setting and complete your data collection, account for any implications of the loss of setting on the results in your final report. Explain the reasons for the loss and the strategies which you implemented to ensure the conditions in the alternative setting were comparable with those originally encountered.

The least attractive option of the three is to abandon your research and down grade the study to pilot study status. This fate is usually reserved for studies in their infancy where insufficient data has been collected to reveal any meaningful findings. If this situation arises, review the data and the procedures used to collect it, and make any amendments which will improve the process or the outcome. Defer the study until a suitable source of data again becomes available.

Disruption of the work force

Depending upon their scale, changes to the composition and/or organisation of the work force in the setting during the course of your study may impact upon the collection of data. For example, in areas where agency or casual pool staff are frequently used, the recruitment of subjects or the interrater reliability of any data collected may be jeopardised. The latter is particularly true if the regular staff have undergone special training to enable them to collect valid and reliable data for you.

Being aware of the staffing profile of the research setting before you implement your project will allow you to assess the impact of a mobile work force on the collection of your data. You will also be in a better position to control the influence of this confounding variable before the reliability of any data is jeopardised. If you anticipate that temporary staff may be supplying data for you, make provision on the data collection form for assessors to indicate whether they are casual or permanent employees. This may enable you to account for any incongruent data which becomes evident during the processing of the results.

Just as the composition of the work force may influence the value of the data, organisational changes imposed on the regular staff may have a similar effect. Change within the organisation which significantly impacts on the designation or duties of the staff (e.g. the implementation of a new career structure or the amalgamation of agencies) will often mean that extraneous activities, including the collection of your data, receive scant attention.

For these reasons, try to avoid settings where any major reorganisation of the work force relevant to your research (e.g. of nurses) is planned. If this is not possible, you will need to wait until the impact of the change has passed, and the staff have become familiar with their new roles before attempting to implement your study. Not to do so can lead to a disappointing return of data. At the very best the collection of your data will be disrupted to some degree. At worst it will simply be suspended—with dire consequences for the study.

Problems with data collection

The problems relating to the collection of data in the research setting can usually be attributed to the relevance of the research problem to the setting or the extra work associated with collecting the data. The strategies outlined here are those which have been successfully used by nurse researchers in the past to maximise the return of data in clinical settings.

Compliance by staff

Requirements seen as a burden. Poor compliance with the requirements of the study will invariably occur when the tasks associated with the research are too time consuming for the staff to perform during a busy shift. Although it was stated in Chapter 5 that the best kind of clinical research does not add substantially to the work load, this is not strictly true. Where a study seeks to substantiate the need for a long-standing procedure, seemingly undertaken for traditional reasons, e.g. the removal of patients' pyjama pants during tonsillectomies (Brown 1993), subjects in the experimental study group will normally have the procedure withheld, thus decreasing the work load. In these kinds of projects, the rate of staff compliance is normally very high with few difficulties being encountered during the data collection phase.

If the tasks associated with your research demand significant extra work, it is likely that they will be deferred until the time becomes available to complete them. It is a sad fact of life however, that although staff may be keen to assist you, the time is never available for them to do so. Consequently precious data collection opportunities may be lost in the wake of other tasks with higher priorities.

Problems related to the extra work load incurred by nurses during the collection of data should be recognised during the pilot study (see Ch. 5). When problems are identified, modifications to the data collection process should be made to eliminate or minimise their impact. Sometimes modification to the process is not possible and you have no alternative but to persevere with the time consuming methods. In this case you might try heightening your profile in the research setting, either by providing feedback on the progress of the study or small rewards for contribution to the data. You may also consider increasing your own contribution to the process or extending the period of time allocated to data collection.

Lack of expertise. If your research requires special expertise to collect the data (e.g. collection of blood), during your reconnaissance visit to the setting, you will need to establish that sufficient staff have the skills to perform the required tasks. If the setting can provide sufficient study subjects but few (or none) of the staff have the expertise to collect the data, organise training sessions to provide the staff who will be involved in the study with the necessary skills to fulfil their role as data collectors. Do this *before* you begin to collect the data.

If the expertise is not available and it is not possible to conduct training sessions, you will need to find an alternative setting where staff have or can acquire the required skills to fulfil the requirements of the project. Alternatively, consider hiring someone to collect the data for you.

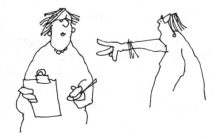

Compliance by subjects

Problems with the collection of data may arise if the subjects are required to continue an experimental or control treatment following discharge from the research setting. In these instances the question which arises most commonly is 'how do you know how compliant patients are, once they are out of the research setting?' If the prescribed treatment contravenes any customs observed by members of specific ethnic, cultural or social groups, you have little chance of achieving compliance by subjects who are members of these groups once they return home. Therefore when compiling your research protocol, it is important that you identify those groups whose cultural beliefs will prohibit them from complying with the requirements of your research and exclude them from the study population.

Assessing compliance by subjects. If your study involves follow up visits to the subject's home, check the residues of lotions and creams, etc. in bottles and tubes. While this is not irrefutable evidence (the contents may have gone down the sink!), it may be your only indication of compliance. If no arrangement for visits exists, but the subject is receiving ongoing treatment from a domiciliary service (e.g. community nurses), enlist their help to make these checks for you.

In many cases a form that can be ticked or initialled following each occasion of treatment can enhance the chances of compliance. The presence of a specially designed form that is *easy to complete* may be enough to remind a subject to comply with the requirements of your study.

Random spot checks on the subject following discharge may also give you an idea of compliance. If you choose this option, you should advise your subjects during recruitment that home visits following discharge are a possibility. When you do call on subjects at home, vary the time and the day of the visit. If your subjects become familiar with any routine you adopt, they may reserve their compliance solely to coincide with the time they anticipate a visit.

As you will never be able to establish absolute proof of subject's compliance with the requirements of the research, accept your results for what they are. Process the data as though all subjects were compliant—unless you know for certain that this was not the case. If you suspect the rate of compliance may have influenced the results (in any way whatsoever), acknowledge the possibility as a limitation of your study.

Uninspiring questionnaires

People usually like to talk about themselves and therefore patients who are bored may enjoy working through a questionnaire to pass the time. Long boring questionnaires, however, will tend to deter members of your sample and contribute to a low response rate. Guidelines for developing a user friendly questionnaire may be found in Chapter 5.

Special groups

For a variety of reasons some subjects will present you with special challenges during data collection. When approaching patients who fall into the categories described below, assess the impact that these factors will have on the collection of your data. If you decide there is no foreseeable risk of jeopardising the quality of the data, proceed as planned. If however, the data is likely to be compromised by proceeding in an unfavourable climate, you should either postpone collection until a more appropriate time or, where circumstances are unlikely to change, exclude the subject from your study.

Subjects who are acutely ill

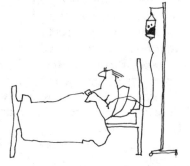

While approval of your research protocol by the IEC will allow you to access patients who may be acutely ill, this sanction will not guarantee that the data collected during the acute phase of an illness will be of sufficient quality to be useful. For example, patients who have undergone lengthy surgical procedures are prone to extreme tiredness in the early post-operative period. They are therefore usually unable to maintain concentration during interviews and other lengthy data collection exercises conducted during this time. Similarly the quality of data provided by patients distracted by pain, breathlessness, nausea or an unfavourable prognosis may also be jeopardised.

For these reasons it is essential when planning studies which require the use of sick patients, that you consider the extent to which the subject's condition may influence his or her ability to co-operate with requirements of the data collection process. If the quality of the data provided is likely to be affected by the subject's condition, you should consider using the medical record rather than attempt a face-to-face confrontation during the acute phase of the patient's illness. If this source will not provide the necessary data, consider accessing an alternative population which can also provide the answers to the research question. If no such alternative exists, consider delaying the collection of data until a time when your subject will be able to co-operate with the requirements of your data collection methods.

As suggested in Chapter 5, if your study involves interaction or intervention in the immediate post-operative phase, obtain the subject's consent pre-operatively. In the immediate post-operative phase, people may refuse to participate in a study because they do not feel well enough to make a decision about the tasks associated with providing the required data. If you obtain consent before surgery, post-operatively you will need only briefly disturb your subject—to re-introduce yourself, remind them of the requirements of the study, confirm their willingness to participate, and all being well, collect your data.

Illiterate subjects

Where subjects appear vague or reluctant to complete a questionnaire, consider the possibility that they may be illiterate. Generally adults or adolescents will not admit to being unable to read and therefore it will be up to you to detect their deficit. Excuses such as 'I don't like filling out forms' or 'I haven't got my glasses' may be an indication of illiteracy. If these reasons are offered as an excuse, suggest conducting the session as an interview. Alternatively, offer to read the questionnaire to the subject, e.g. 'Is it easier if I read it out for you?'

Collecting data from difficult subjects

While most of the data collected in face-to-face encounters will be obtained from pleasant, co-operative subjects, occasionally you may come into contact with subjects who, because of their aggression or other antisocial characteristics, may unsettle you.

When approaching subjects whom you perceive to have the potential to present you with difficulties, introduce yourself and break the ice using small talk. During this warm up phase, let the other person set the pace and topic of conversation and/or let off steam as the need arises. This will allow him or her to gradually gain confidence in you (and your ability). Remind yourself that any manifestation of aggressive behaviour maybe merely a facade which is symptomatic of an underlying frustration, and that simply making the time to sit and talk to the patient may be enough to dissipate any manifest aggression.

If during the course of this preliminary conversation a problem is mentioned which you are in a position to solve yourself (or delegate to someone else to do so), offer to fix it. Reserve offers like this however, for small problems with simple short term solutions. Under no circumstances should you make a commitment which you *cannot fulfil* or (worse still) have *no intention* of carrying out.

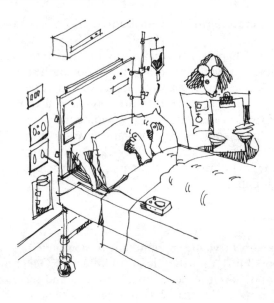

Before you attempt to seek consent for participation in your study, try to gain enough rapport with the person to feel comfortable in their presence. Be aware however, that to get this far may entail several visits. The amount of effort you expend to recruit one subject will depend largely on the size of the study population and how precious each person is to the study. If you have access to a large pool of potential subjects you may be able to avoid approaching the most difficult subjects. Unless your population sample is extremely small, it will add nothing to the study (or your morale) if you doggedly pursue really unpleasant individuals.

Even though you may ultimately gain consent for participation from these people, if it is obtained under silent protest there may be retribution—in the form of incomplete, irrational or sabotaged data. Where this possibility exists, it is not worth the effort entailed and you should not pursue the recruitment of this type of individual. If you choose not to include people who satisfy the inclusion criteria, acknowledge the omission, and the reasons for it in your research report.

Language and cultural differences

Coping with language differences

While it is true that it is often easier to exclude non-English speaking subjects, you should think carefully before deciding to do so. It is highly likely that study populations drawn from public hospitals will include some members of ethnic minorities. While this may not influence the collection of objective data, which is not open to interpretation, in studies where it is thought that ethnic origin might have a bearing on the data (particularly in the light of generalisability), you may miss important information by excluding ethnic minorities from your sample.

If your study is dependant on fluency in the English language, you will need to ensure that your subjects have either sufficient mastery of the language themselves to enable them to interpret the data collection instruments correctly, or the potential to do so with the assistance of an interpreter.

Be aware that some people who claim to understand English may have difficulty interpreting colloquial phrases or statements out of context. Questions which offer multiple choices which express feelings may also cause problems. For example statements such as 'I feel worried' can give rise to feelings of insecurity or confusion (e.g. should I feel worried?).

Documentation. If you include non-English speaking subjects in your study, prepare comprehensive information sheets and get these and your consent forms translated into the language used by the ethnic groups who make up a substantial proportion of your study population. While this may be an expensive exercise, it is well worth the money if you have a number of significant subgroups, as it minimises the language barrier during recruitment. Be certain to pilot these documents, to ensure their context and presentation are correct, before using them on a large scale.

Interpreters. Ideally, when recruiting subjects with non-English speaking backgrounds, you should take an interpreter from a recognised service with you on at least one of your two recruitment visits. On the first visit leave the information with the subject to read at their leisure. In a few days return with an interpreter to answer questions and collect the signed consent form. If you choose not to use an interpreter, it will be up to you to assess whether the subject understands you sufficiently to both give his or her informed consent and participate meaningfully in the study.

If you recruit subjects whose ability to comprehend the questions may be suspect, the use of an interpreter during the collection of your data is recommended. For studies where large numbers of subjects from non-English speaking backgrounds are involved, this can be expensive. If the cost prohibits the use of interpreters, you will need to ensure your questions are short, to the point and not open to any degree of misinterpretation. In particular, avoid the use of jargon or colloquial language which may confuse a subject whose first language is not English.

On no account should you rely on relatives, or a staff member (e.g. nurse, cleaner) who speaks the language, to assist you with recruitment or the collection of your data. They may inadvertently exert subtle pressure on a subject to participate in the study, or introduce bias into the explanation during an interview. If you cannot understand what is being asked of the subject, you will not appreciate any influence being used to persuade a person to participate. Likewise, if the data is not being accurately interpreted, you will not be aware of any discrepancies being reported.

Coping with cultural or social differences

Where members of minority groups (e.g. homosexuals or ethnic or racial minorities) are to form part of your sample, you will need to do some extra homework when designing your data collection tool. It is important to your credibility as a legitimate researcher that you become aware of any social or cultural taboos which may apply before you inadvertently plough in with offensive questions or unacceptable requests during data collection. The success of your interaction with members of minority groups during data collection will depend on it.

For example, in some ethnic groups certain topics may not be broached by females. Therefore, if you are female and envisage including male members of a minority group, who may not regard questions coming from you as being acceptable, consider co-opting a male of cultural background similar to that of the subjects to collect the data. If this is not possible and problems do arise, omit the inappropriate questions when interviewing members of relevant groups and acknowledge the deletion as a limitation of the study.

On no account should you knowingly pursue a line of questioning that transgresses the cultural mores of the study participants. Your persistence may ultimately stifle the provision of any meaningful data from the individual, who loses all respect for you as a credible researcher.

Sensitive topics

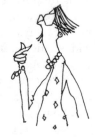

Like nurses, patients need to trust the credibility of the researcher before they will divulge sensitive information about themselves for research purposes. Therefore, if your study requires the disclosure of personal details, it will be up to you to establish that trust during your initial contact with the members of the study population. Full disclosure of the research requirements (and a willingness to share some personal details about yourself) during recruitment is one way of establishing a subject's trust in you. In itself however, this may not be enough to allay any lingering misgivings about participation. You should therefore reinforce the provisions for maintaining confidentiality during the distribution of questionnaires or before beginning any interview.

The ultimate success of an interview will depend largely on the degree of trust which exists between you and your subject, and your ability to set him or her at ease while discussing sensitive issues. In this regard, *a private, comfortable interview setting is a must*. It is also essential that *you* become totally at ease with the subject matter *before* you attempt to ask personal questions which may cause subjects to become embarrassed. Remember too that your chances of collecting the required information will be enhanced if you can demonstrate the links between any personal questions and the stated aims of the research. It is therefore recommended that you probe the more sensitive issues through the use of questions which are in a logical order and which progressively expand on topics covered in previous questions.

Conclusion

Careful planning is the key to conducting successful research in the clinical setting and most of the difficulties described in this chapter can be minimised or eliminated if you can answer 'yes' to the following questions before you attempt to implement your study.

- Is the problem being investigated relevant to this setting?
- Does the study have the potential to improve patient care?
- Can the setting provide at least twice the required number of subjects in the time allocated for the study?
- Is the setting expected to be available for the entire data collection period?
- Do the staff in the setting have the skills required to perform the tasks associated with the study?
- Will the staff be able to perform the tasks associated with the collection of data without adding significantly to their work load?
- Can the identified confounding variables be minimised or eliminated?

If the answer to any of these questions is no, it is likely that some administrative difficulties will be experienced during the collection of data. You should therefore assess the likely impact of any identified potential or actual problems on the rate of recruitment or the quality of the data *before* you implement your study. Matching a relevant problem to an appropriate setting and completing a study which brings about an improvement in patient care will generally bring with it a great deal of personal satisfaction. To implement a study in the face of the adverse conditions discussed in this chapter however, is suicidal and will give rise to much frustration and anxiety during its conduct. As such, this course is not recommended.

REFERENCES

Brown G 1993 The sacred cow contest. Canadian Nurse Jan 31–33

7. Managing quantitative data

Pat Rapley

Although quantitative data can be easily prepared for analysis by computer, the pitfalls in the process are numerous. The purpose of this chapter therefore is to outline the strategies which have been shown to minimise the loss of data through poor compliance with the data collection instrument, and describe the processes associated with the preparation of quantitative data for computer analysis.

Quantitative data can be both meaningful, e.g. temperature, age in years or weight in kilograms, or in the case of syllabic statements which need to be converted into numbers for processing, meaningless. For example the variable sex may be assigned two numbers, 1 for female and 2 for male. These values are meaningless as they are arbitrarily assigned. Similarly the Likert scale is an example of numbers without value. Unlike the previous example however, the numbers assigned to represent degrees of agreement or disagreement do represent an order from 1 to 5 or 1 to 7.

Just as there are many data collection techniques, there are also more than 180 statistical software packages that can be used to analyse data on main-frame computers—in addition to more than 40 others designed for use on personal computers (Hannah 1987). Whether the statistical package is Mystat, SPSS (Statistical Packages for the Social Sciences), SAS (Statistical Analysis System) or some other statistical software, the instrument to collect the data must be designed so as to maximise the return of valid data. In addition, the accuracy of the data needs to checked following its collection and entry.

Explanation of terms

Case: all the data collected from one subject is called a case. Each case will consist of several variables.

Field: the number of columns assigned to each variable. For example, the answer to the question 'how many years since registration' uses a two column field. As some of the subjects would have registered more than 9 years ago, two columns are needed for numbers greater than 9 and equal to or less than 99. It is unlikely however, that three columns would ever be required, as subjects who registered more than 99 years ago are extremely rare.

119

File: a file can be likened to a manilla folder in a drawer. The disk which contains the file is the drawer. As each subset of information is often stored as one entity in a file of its own, you may need to create a data file and a command file in the same way that you create a text file using a word processor. Depending on the statistical package however, it may be possible to create one file for both the data and the commands to analyse it.

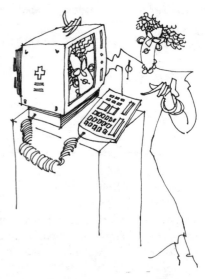

The *data* file consists of columns and rows of numbers entered according to the questionnaire design. The *command* file enables the statistical analyses you require to be carried out—usually in a fraction of the time it would take by pen or calculator. Before the computer can execute the commands however, it has to know the location (column number) of the data to be analysed. An error in data entry, either incorrect number in correct column or a correct number in an incorrect column, can result in an incorrect analysis. When you multiply the number of cases (subjects) by the number of columns used for each case, it becomes evident that the potential for error is great.

An *output* file is created when data is processed in accordance with the program's commands. As it will contain the results of the statistical tests you requested, it is the file you need to write up your research findings.

Record: each horizontal line of numbers in a data file is a record. For large questionnaires you may need to allow for more than one record (line) per case (subject). If more than one record is needed, a record identifier column will be required.

Scale: set of sequential responses or a diagram used to measure an abstract concept, e.g. Likert, semantic differential or visual analogue (VAS) scales.

Values: each response in a questionnaire is entered into the data file (coded) as a number. These numbers are called values. Missing values are blank spaces in the record where a value was expected.

Variable: a characteristic or attribute to be measured in the study.

Questionnaire design

Although questionnaires are used extensively as data collection instruments, the information they provide does not always live up to the researcher's expectations. This is because questionnaire design is a skill which is said to have been mastered only when the maximum amount of useful information is received from a minimum number of questions. Simplicity and brevity are the keys to maximising the return of valid data from your population sample. Respondents generally appreciate questions which are easy to understand and a questionnaire which takes only a short time to complete.

Putting the question

It is essential that the data collection instrument provides for the collection of precise information about the variables likely to influence the results of your study. Therefore when formulating your questions, always keep the aims of the research in mind. It will assist you to determine whether the questions have the potential to yield the data required to answer your research question. The so called fishing expeditions which seek information irrelevant to the scope of the study are not regarded as acceptable by ethics committees, subjects or experienced researchers. As such, they should be avoided at all times.

Include only those questions which fall within the known knowledge base of your study population. If you are unsure about the ability of a subject to answer, include a 'don't know' option in the list of responses to multiple choice questions. It will help to eliminate the possibility of missing values or incorrect responses (due to guesses).

Group all questions about a similar theme (e.g. demographic details) together. Focus each question on one concept at a time. Two-part questions which may require a different response for each part (e.g. do anxiety and nausea influence the pain threshold?) tend to confuse the respondent. While leaving the space blank will solve the dilemma for the subject, this is missing data and the gap may necessitate extra work for you later.

Phrase your questions so that they encourage the respondents to think about each question. Questions which alternate between positive and negative statements may eliminate the tendency for respondents to fall into a constant (or donkey) response. Therefore, if you can mix the statement biases without jeopardising the clarity of the question, do so—but be sure to provide a clear indication of the topic in the sentence stem of each new question.

For questions which require a scaled response, as the Likert type scale shown below, the literature is divided as to whether you should offer an odd or even number of alternatives. For example:

```
Q13a  I enjoy coming to work (circle one number)
        always                          1
        frequently                      2
        seldom                          3
        never                           4
```

or, alternatively:

Q13b I enjoy coming to work (circle one number)

always	1
frequently	2
uncertain	3
seldom	4
never	5

By providing an even number of alternatives (as in Q13a of this example), your respondents will be forced to decide between a positive or negative response (Abdellah & Levine 1986). You will also have the advantage of being able to collapse the data into two groups if necessary. While this reduction of the data will result in a loss of detail, it can facilitate your analysis by enabling you to determine the broad trends evident in the data. If you need a sensitive instrument that will detect the small differences between the respondents, you will need to include more options, perhaps a 7, 8 or 9 point scale. The choice of how sensitive to make your question is ultimately yours. Be wary however of offering too many alternatives to a small study sample. It will spread the responses too thinly and cause problems with data analysis.

By contrast, if you choose to use an existing questionnaire, the questions would be coded according to the author's instructions. That is, if you were interested in the Self-efficacy Scale developed by Sherer et al (1982), you would need to seek approval to use it. Once approved, you would need to use their format. For more detailed advice on questionnaire design, you should consult any of the excellent books available on the subject such as Converse and Presser (1986), Dillman (1978) Sudman and Bradburn (1982).

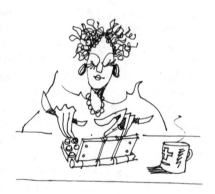

Order of questions

It is your choice as to whether you begin or end with questions relating to the characteristics of the sample or demographic profile (such as age, gender, educational level, income, job classification, etc.). As these questions require little deliberation by the respondent, if placed at the beginning of the document, they often allow the respondent to move easily into the body of the questionnaire. On the debit side however, these questions often require personal information which the subject may regard as an invasion of privacy. In these cases (if you see the form again), you may find these and other questions left unanswered.

Using a diagram to put the question

A 100 mm vertical or horizontal Visual Analogue Scale (VAS) is commonly used to obtain information about very subjective or abstract concepts (such as pain or anxiety). Each end of the line has right angle stops and is annotated with the extreme descriptors of the concept being measured (Fig. 7.1). During data collection the subject is asked to place a cross at the point on the line which indicates the quality or intensity of the concept being measured. The distance measured from the left of a horizontal line or one end of the vertical line then becomes the score for the variable.

Formatting your questionnaire for computer analysis

Column numbers. Ease of data entry from the questionnaire to the data file is directly related to the questionnaire format or layout. As the person entering the values in the computer needs to refer constantly to the field of column numbers, these are usually placed on the right hand side of the page in close proximity to the entries to be made by the subjects (see Fig. 7.2). This makes them easier to read during data entry.

Field size. The allocation of a field to each variable should include enough columns for the type of response expected. Begin by allocating sufficient columns for the case (subject's) identifier number, and then a column for the record identifier number as required. If the sample size is expected to be no more than 99, then a two column field for the ID or identification number will suffice. A sample of more than 99 but equal to or less than 999 will require a three column field. In the latter case the field for a record would then be column four. A one column field for the record will give you nine records or nine lines of data at 80 columns per line.

Field size for each question (variable) will depend upon the type of response. Where only one number is to be circled, allocate only one column. However, where subjects can circle more than one number to answer the question, one column per possible response is required. If two digit numbers are required in the response, a field of two columns is required.

If you are prepared to allow for more than one response to a question, make this clear in the instruction and allow sufficient columns. Figure 7.3 is an example of a multiple response question using a six column field. There is however a problem with this layout. See *Accounting for blank spaces in a record* and compare Figure 7.3 to Figure 7.4.

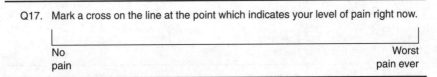

Q17. Mark a cross on the line at the point which indicates your level of pain right now.

No
pain

Worst
pain ever

Fig. 7.1 Example of a 100 mm visual analogue scale (VAS) to measure pain.

		Col
ID number	☐☐	1–2
Record	☐	3

Q1.   What is your gender?
(Please circle one number)

Female	1	
Male	2	4

Q2.   What is your age in years?
(Please fill in boxes: whole numbers only)   ☐☐   5–6

Q3.   How many years since initial registration?
(Please fill in boxes: whole numbers only)   ☐☐   7–8

Q4.   What is your current position?
(Please circle one number)

Enrolled Nurse	1	
Registered Nurse	2	
Clinical Nurse	3	
Clinical Nurse Specialist	4	9

Q5.   Do you believe all nurses are caring people? (Please circle one number)

Yes	1	(Go to Q6)	10
No	2	(Go to Q9)	

Fig. 7.2 Example of questionnaire format

Length of record. Another formatting question to consider when designing the questionnaire is the length of the record. If you want to keep the entire record visible on the screen, you will need to limit each record to 80 columns. An appropriate place to change to the next record, is after a set of related questions—even if this occurs at column 69. If the next section of the questionnaire has 23 related questions, it is easier to have them all in the one record by changing to record two at the start of the questions.

Q14.   Which of the following journals have you read in the last month?
(circle all relevant numbers)

Advances in Nursing Science	1	40
Aust J. Advanced Nursing	2	41
Contemporary Nurse	3	42
Nursing Research	4	43
Nursing Science Quarterly	5	44
Topics in Clinical Nursing	6	45

Fig. 7.3 Example of a multiple response question using six single column fields.

Data preparation and organisation

Checking the data

Before the entry of data begin, someone needs to check the data collection forms for errors and omissions. Although pre-testing your instrument should detect some ambiguities in the questions, blank spaces will still occur.

Accounting for blank spaces in a record

The number of missing values or blank spaces needs to be assessed before data analysis begins as they influence some statistical tests. Blank spaces due to non-compliance can result from the subject's indecision, refusal to answer or lack of knowledge, and are legitimate missing values. Also, inability of the research assistant to obtain the information or a breakdown in the monitoring equipment can result in missing values.

All blank column spaces are however not necessarily missing values. For example, questions designed to have more than one response such as Q14 (Fig 7.3) will generate blank columns. The field for such questions is large to enable multiple responses to the question. The six columns assigned to that question may have any three of the six cues used by most respondents, leaving three columns blank. If a yes/no response for each cue was used (Fig 7.4), then all columns theoretically would be used with no missing values. However you design the instrument, the computer may still need to be told the difference between missing data and blank columns. This problem also applies to the filter questions discussed below.

As part of the data preparation process, you may wish to assign different numbers to the varying types of missing values: 0 'no value recorded', 9 'refused to answer'. Most statistical packages have default procedures or options for handling cases with missing values. You should check the relevant manual for specific requirements of the software package you plan to use.

Q14. Which of the following journals have you read in the last month? (circle one number for each journal)			
	yes	no	
Advances in Nursing Science	1	2	40
Aust J. Advanced Nursing	1	2	41
Contemporary Nurse	1	2	42
Nursing Research	1	2	43
Nursing Science Quarterly	1	2	44
Topics in Clinical Nursing	1	2	45

Fig 7.4 Example of a multiple response question using six single column fields that will not generate blank responses in the record.

It will be up to you to determine the importance of the missing data. When making your decision consider the following questions:

- Without this data, will the subject have to be withdrawn from the study?
- Can the code sheet be used to follow up individuals again?
- Should a special code be used for the 'no response' category?

The answers to these questions will need to be determined before a professional data entry service can start processing your forms.

Recording errors

Responses need also to be checked for errors in recording. For example, subjects may circle two numbers, when only one is wanted (and allowed for in the field). As you have no way of knowing which number has priority, neither can be used. Conversely, when two columns have been allowed, but the subject incorrectly uses only one. For example:

		Col.
Q3.	How many years since your initial registration?	
	(Please fill in boxes: whole numbers only) ☐☐	7–8

The correct way to complete the boxes is to place a zero in the first box for numbers less than 10. If however, a subject puts a 2 in the first box (column 7), and the entry coder does likewise, the computer will probably still read it as 02. To be sure though, the source material should be checked for these and other errors or omissions before data entry commences.

Data entry

The creation of a data file requires uninterrupted attention to detail. Taking the time to eliminate errors at this stage will save time later and ensure that results are correct. It is necessary to ensure that the number corresponding to the subject's answer is recorded correctly, as well as recorded in the correct column of the data file: correct number, correct column. Unfortunately, a spell-check equivalent does not exist to detect entry errors. There are however ways to minimise mistakes incurred during data entry, i.e.:

- ensure the questionnaire is set up to facilitate ease of data entry;
- use a professional data collation (entry) service;
- use two people, one to enter while the other checks.

Inspecting the data file print-out

Although the strategies listed above will facilitate the accurate entry of data, it is also wise to check the data file and the subsequent print-out of frequencies obtained for each variable before commencing your data analysis.

Visual comparison. Visual comparisons of the data print-out are easier with a fixed format questionnaire, but only really aberrant numbers will stand out and be queried as errors. Specifically, this involves inspecting each column (vertical row) of the data file print-out using a ruler or a template. For example, if the answer to Q1 in column 4 in Figure 7.2, has a choice of two numbers (female 1, male 2), then by placing a ruler alongside column 4 of the print-out, any numbers other than those expected will be readily seen.

Running frequency counts

Frequency counts for each variable can be ordered once the data has been entered into a data file and the command file has been created. Since you know how many subjects are in the sample tested and the approximate major demographic breakdown of males/females, age groups, etc., inspection of the print-out from a frequencies command should there-fore match your expectations.

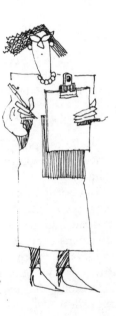

Numbers that deviate from the expected for any one variable can be identified and a search conducted for the source of the error. It is, however, only those numbers that lie at the extremes of the expected range that are likely to be questioned.

Variations could indicate an error in the data entry process, or the command you used to obtain the frequencies, or your expectations. A process of elimination is then needed to ensure the data are correct.

Data transformation

Data preparation also requires that some values for a variable be changed before analysis. Although this sounds a bit like cheating, it is both legal and necessary.

Extending the boundaries by grouping data. The object of analysing data is to answer the research question. Therefore groups formed by collapsing the ratio or interval data into categorical data (nominal) should only be created to achieve this end. For example, continuous data collected in response to the question 'What is your age?', can be regrouped using the following SPSS command according to a predetermined definition of young adult, middle aged and old:

Recode age(18 thru 35=1)(36 thru 60=2)(61 thru hi=3) into agegr.

In this way, the recode command can be used to convert the continuous data associated with the variable 'age' into three nominal categories of the now new variable 'agegr', without losing the original data of the variable age. The choice of limits for each variable group can be determined from those used in previous research cited in the literature, or arbitrarily assigned after examination of the original frequency results.

It is also possible to form groups on the basis of two variable values. That is, using a type of 'If' command, the groups can be defined on the basis of gender as well as age, or any other two variables. In SPSS this command is:

If sex = 2 and age GE 18 and LE 35 agegr = 1

This command is then repeated for each of the new groups to be created. The result is that the new age groups formed are as before, but are also single sex as the computer only selects on sex=2.

A new variable can also be created using logical expressions such as 'Let', and 'If...Then let'. In Mystat the command is:

If age=<40 Then let newgroup=1 (Mystat, version 2.0, 1988).

While the possibilities to regroup and extend the data are endless, the research question/s to be answered should determine any regrouping of data.

Recoding data. Recoding data is a necessity for some analyses. A typical example of the need to recode would be the positively and negatively worded statements in a Likert scale. See Table 7.1 for an example of two questions (items) in a Likert scale. Beside each of the statements in the questionnaire are numbers to be circled. The numbers are graded in order, 1 to 5 or 1 to 7 equating with degree of agreement or disagreement with the statements. To avoid an answering bias, these numbers stay constant regardless of the direction of the statements. A recode type command is used to restore the order. That is, if 5 equates with strongly agree (SA) in a positively worded statement, then the same person is likely to circle 1 for strongly disagree (SD) in a negatively worded statement. If 5 = SA, then high scores would represent positive attitudes, and vice versa.

Table 7.1 Example of a Likert scale layout for two items

Value statement	SD	D	?	A	SA
+ nursing care should be based on research findings	1	2	3	4	5
- research is not relevant to a practice based discipline	1	2	3	4	5

Key: +/- signs to indicate bias of question explained in this chapter (not to be included in actual questionnaire).

Table 7.1 illustrates the point. In this example, the addition of 5 + 1 would not represent the true numerical value of that person's attitude to the variable. Therefore, a command is used to recode specific questions (either the negatively worded or the positively worded) so that 1 = 5, 2 = 4, 4 = 2, 5 = 1. In this way the person would now score 5 + 5. The recode procedure is quite simple and should be explained in the manual of any statistical package.

Transforming filter questions. Filter questions are used to direct respondents to appropriate next questions. That is, the respondent's answer will determine which question they should answer next. The typical scenario is:

Q5.   Do you believe all nurses are caring people? (circle one number)
       Yes   1   (Go to Q6)
       No   2   (Go to Q9)

Analysis of this data can be preceded by a command that selects the subjects (cases) who circled 1 for yes (the filter question), and their answers to the following related questions:

        temporary
        select if Q5=1
        NPAR TESTS corr Q1 Q2 Q3 Q6 Q7 Q8.

If using SPSS, the *temporary* command ensures that the *select if* command only applies to the next analysis ordered. That is, only those subjects who answered yes for Q5 will have a Pearson's rank order correlation analysis of their answers in relation to Q1 (gender), Q2 (age), Q3 (registration), and Q6 to 8 (which expands on why they consider nurses to be caring people). This will avoid the analysis of blanks generated by Q6 to 8 for the group who answered no to the filter question. Most other statistical packages have an equivalent temporary type command or procedure that only applies to the next analysis. Similarly, the exact wording of the command for a non-parametric analysis, or indeed any analysis command, will depend upon the statistical package used. 'NPAR TESTS' is the specific SPSS command for non-parametric tests of correlation.

Processing the data

Processing the data includes reporting the demographic data to set the scene, followed by the inferential statistics according to the research question or hypothesis statements.

Profiling study participants

Analysis of data used to set the scene and describe the sample is referred to as descriptive statistics. When inferences, from the sample data, about a target population are to be made it is important to have given as much background information as possible. Specifically, the demographic and or socioeconomic data could include such variables as age, gender, marital status, number of dependent children, years since obtaining initial nursing registration, highest educational qualification, present position. The choice of the specific demographic and socioeconomic variables is important as they are used to draw a verbal picture of the sample, and the subgroups within the sample, to enable comparisons with previous and future studies.

More specifically, the text reports means and standard deviations for symmetrical interval and ratio data (the distance between any two numbers on the scale that are equal and of known size). The median however, is used with standard deviation for skewed interval and ratio data. Percentages are used for ordinal (graded syllabic data) and nominal data (categories of a given variable). Graphs, pie charts, histograms or other tabular representations of data are also used to stress significant or interesting results. Table 7.2 gives an example of nominal (sex) and ratio (age) data.

Considerable attention to detail is needed at this stage to ensure that the figures reported in both the text and a table are the same. The decision as to the degree of detail in both text and tabular form will depend upon the style guide of the journal to which you plan to submit your findings. See the section on graphical presentation of data (below) for further discussion on this point.

Inferential choices

While the purpose of research is to seek an answer, the accuracy of the answer is dependent upon the appropriateness of the statistical analysis. Although parametric tests are more powerful than non-parametric tests, they are not always the most appropriate type of analysis.

'Inferential statistics...allow investigators to reach conclusions about relationships among variables or differences between groups in populations from samples.' (Thomas 1990). An inference is made about the probability of making a correct or incorrect decision about the target population based on a sample of that population. For example, the finding about occupa-

Table 7.2 Percentages (%), Means (M) and Standard Deviations (SD) of demographic data by diabetes type (Iddm/Niddm)

Variable	IDDM (n=49)			NIDDM (n=48)		
	%	M	SD	%	M	SD
Sex (male)	59.2			47.9		
Age (years)		37.6	15.5		60.0	12.9

Key: Iddm   Insulin dependent diabetes mellitus.
      Niddm   Non insulin dependent diabetes mellitus.

tional stress in registered nurses is more likely to be correctly generalised to the whole registered nurse population if a random sample of all RNs in Australia was used in the study. Inferences about the total can be made from a well chosen few.

The choice of inferential test will firstly involve the determination of whether the assumption of normality can be met.

Assumptions of normality. Use of parametric statistical procedures, such as t-tests, ANOVA or Pearson's product moment correlation, assumes that the data set has been derived from a normal or approximately normal population. Amongst other things, a normal distribution is characterised by the fact that the distribution of scores represents a bell shaped curve, each measurement falls somewhere along a continuum (continuous measurement) and the scores are symmetrically distributed around the mean (Knapp 1985).

Therefore, another reason to produce frequency distributions with your first command is to check the distribution of each variable about normality. Histograms and plot commands can also be used to determine if the characteristic bell shaped curve of a normal distribution is present for each of the variables of interest.

Non-parametric tests, such as Spearman's rank order correlation, are therefore generally used for the asymmetric data set and nominal or ordinal variables. For more information on parametric or non-parametric tests, a specific statistical text should be consulted as there are some important exemptions to this very brief guide. In both Knapp (1985) and Shott (1990) a decision tree algorithm has been included to assist you with the selection of an appropriate method of statistical analysis based on the research design. The decision tree is useful in that it provides a step wise series of questions about the research design. By answering each step, the reader is led to another level of questions, resulting in the specific tests appropriate for the study.

Level of measurement. The choice of statistical test is also determined by the sample size and the level of measurement. The main aim is to preserve as much interval and or ratio data as possible. The less refined levels of measurement include ordinal and nominal values which traditionally have been restricted to the less powerful non-parametric procedures. This convention, however, is less rigidly applied today (Thomas 1990).

Ratio or interval data format in the instrument design is therefore preferable. If, for instance, a correlation between age and some other variable is required, the instrument should include boxes or a space for the person's actual age. Usually a 'age in years only' statement is used, and if necessary, specific computer commands can be used later to collapse the ratio data into appropriate categories.

Graphical presentation of data

As numerical data in a paragraph can be quite hard to read, judicious use of tables (columns of numbers) and figures (histogram, bar chart, pie chart) to summarise large pieces of statistical information can be useful. Advances in word processing packages and the increasingly user friendly statistical packages mean that you can produce tables and figures with relative ease. If you are submitting the work to a publisher, however, there may be other considerations.

Apart from the additional space requirements for tables or figures, they are also more expensive to prepare and produce. In particular, the variety and complexity of figure formats makes them even more expensive than tables to produce.

Once a decision has been made to use a graphical presentation, ensure that:

- headings are brief but explanatory;
- all symbols and abbreviations are explained in a key; and
- all elements are easily read.

Preferably the finished product will fit across the width of the page without the reader having to turn the page sideways, as this can be very annoying.

As the American Psychological Association (APA 1987) guide states, 'an informative table supplements—it does not duplicate—the text.'. The text should explain the main points of the table, highlighting those results relevant to your reason for writing. Many journals (e.g. *Nursing Research* and the *Australian Journal of Advanced Nursing*) express a similar view. If you are however considering submitting a report to a specific journal, it is advisable to obtain a style guide from the publisher (see Ch. 9), as each journal has specific styles of presentation.

Table 7.2 illustrates the essential information for a title and use of a key for abbreviations. The title should indicate the sample or subgroup, type of statistical test applied and the variables being reported.

In this example, all demographic variables are listed and the relevant statistics placed in the appropriate column. The inclusion of the (n = 49) indicates to the reader that IDDM consists of a subgroup of 49 cases. Abbreviations used in the list, other than the commonly accepted ones, can be explained in a key placed at the end of the table. Similarly, a notation at the end will suffice to indicate the p value for any statistically significant results marked by a symbol. While in the past it has been customary to asterisk significant findings and provide an explanatory key (* = p < .05), more recently the practice of specifying the actual p values has gained popularity.

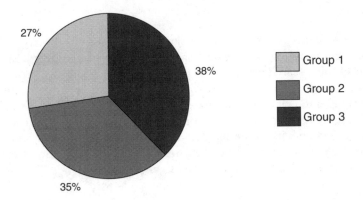

27%

38%

Group 1

Group 2

Group 3

35%

Fig. 7.5 Example of a three group pie chart

The same principles apply for the labelling of a figure, although the convention is to put the title (caption) below the figure and the key (legend) within the figure axis area (APA 1987) as in the pie chart, Figure 7.5.

Choosing the right graphics

Graphic presentation of frequency data, using bar charts, histograms or pie charts, can often be used to illustrate a point more strongly than words or a table. For example, the circle of the pie chart (Figure 7.5) represents 100% of the sample on some variable, each segment of the pie being the percentage value for each subgroup of the variable. It is the simplest way of summarising a variable that only has a small number of distinct values.

Alternatively, a bar chart or histogram can be used to illustrate the point. A bar chart can be used as a graphical representation of a frequency table in which the many values (continuous level data) have been grouped into intervals and the number of cases within each interval then counted. For example, the ages of registered nurses in a sample can be grouped into five-year intervals of 21–25, 26–30, 31–35, etc. A bar chart can also be used to compare related nominal level data such as the number of cases in each of the religious groups of a sample. A bar chart does not have to have an underlying order to the values. There is no order implied in a list of religious groups; they exist and each of us usually nominates allegiance to one or perhaps none.

Conversely, the histogram, which joins the midpoint or middle value of the interval, suggests an order with adjacent values of the variable. It would therefore be appropriate for a histogram to be constructed for the age groups mentioned, but not for the religious groups.

Conclusion

Having made the decision to undertake nursing research, the organisation and processing of quantitative data should be no more daunting than other aspects of the research process. It is hoped that this chapter will help you to design a questionnaire capable of yielding useful data, provide some ideas and strategies to ensure the accurate entry of the data to be processed and offer some useful data transformation techniques to organise your data.

In conjunction with other chapters in this book, the information on data analysis and presentation should ensure a comprehensive and clear summation of the findings of quantitative research studies.

REFERENCES

Abdellah F, Levine E 1986 Better patient care through nursing research, 3rd edn. Macmillan, New York
APA 1987 Publication manual of the American Psychological Association, 3rd edn. American Psychological Association, Washington DC, p 84, p 103
Converse J M, Presser S 1986 Survey questions: handcrafting the standardised questionnaire (quantitative applications in the social sciences series No 63). Sage, Beverley Hills
Dillman D A 1978 Mail and telephone surveys: the total design method. John Wiley, New York
Hannah K 1987 Uses for computers in nursing research. Recent Advances in Nursing 17(2):186–202
Knapp R 1985 Basic statistics for nurses, 2nd edn. John Wiley, New York, p 80
Sherer M, Maddux J, Mercandante B et al 1982 Self efficacy scales: construction and validation. Psychological Reports 51:663–671
Shott S 1990 Statistics for health professionals. W B Saunders, Philadelphia
Sudman S, Bradburn N M 1982 Asking questions. Jossey-Bass, San Francisco
Thomas B 1990 Nursing research: an experiential approach. C V Mosby, St Louis

8. Managing qualitative data

Robin Watts

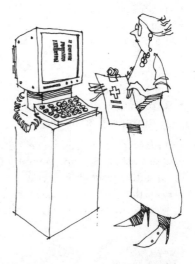

You have completed and transcribed a dozen of the 30 interviews scheduled for your study. Even at this early stage it is likely that you are beginning to feel overwhelmed, both physically, and figuratively, by rapidly mounting stacks of computer paper that contain the precious information collected during these sessions. While the thought of keeping track of your progress with the interview schedules and the processing of the transcripts may be somewhat daunting in itself, this vital aspect of the data collection phase is but only one part of the picture. Somehow, out of the mountain of print outs, you will also have to extract themes and identify the elements required by the type of qualitative method you have employed to address your research question. On their own, each of these tasks can be somewhat arduous. Together they can appear formidable enough to find yourself wishing you had stayed with the number crunching approach of quantitative research.

Don't panic. You are not alone and there are ways out of the maze. I doubt if there is one person who has served an apprenticeship in qualitative methods who hasn't experienced these sorts of feelings. Order can be achieved out of the seeming chaos and the required answers produced. Although each qualitative method has some different requirements, and each individual finds certain strategies more useful than others, the following systematic process, which I developed when faced with these problems may provide ideas as to how to organise and process qualitative data. The examples of processes described here are drawn from a study I conducted in relation to public participation in the health care system (Watts 1992). It may be of assistance to you, if, while you are reading through this chapter, you modify these ideas to fit your research.

Data management

The easiest way of managing your data is to ensure that you always keep track of where you are in terms of the various sets of data you are collecting from different sources. When I was faced with the problem of significant amounts of rapidly accumulating information, I designed a number of data management documents to help me organise and monitor the data collection, generation and analyses processes for each group and respondent participating in the study. These documents are described here and consist of:

- record of contact;
- data processing record;
- data collection log;
- contact summary form;
- document record;
- master sheet;
- exploratory matrices; and
- confirmatory matrices.

The two matrices were based on formats developed by Miles and Huberman (1984) and Marsh (1990). Although these documents may not be directly applicable to your study, their general layout may give you some idea of the kind of records which will enable you to successfully keep track of your progress during the collection of your data.

Record of contact

As I was dealing with a number of very different organisations and individuals, establishing access was a real challenge. A specific approach, often involving a tortuous process to gain entry, needed to be designed for each group and individual. In order to have a handy reference to remind me of where I was at in the process, I drew up a 'method of access' form for each organisation, group or individual participant. On this form I recorded the following information:

- the individuals contacted and the dates contact was made;
- the results of these contacts;
- the subsequent actions to be undertaken;
- the person responsible for taking these actions; and
- the dates by which the actions were to be completed.

I made a habit of checking through these forms on a regular basis to jog my memory and keep the study flowing smoothly. In that way, no element in the study was overlooked for too long.

Data generation

Once you begin collecting data, you will be faced with the problem of managing the rapidly increasing volume of information coming from a variety of different sources. As each interview is completed, a process with numerous phases is set in motion. To keep everything advancing in an organised manner can be real challenge, particularly if your study is just one of a number of demands on your time.

As a general rule, as your data collection gains momentum, each of the preceding interview transcripts should be at a different stage in that process. You don't want to end up with a large number of interview tapes that still have to be transcribed when you suddenly have some spare time, but nothing ready to begin analysing!

Transcribing taped interviews

Before proceeding with the description of documents, it is worth making a note of those points which may assist you with the transcription of audio-taped interviews. Transcriptions should be done on a computer using the same word processing program for all of the transcriptions, rather than on a typewriter. This approach facilitates the use of a computer software package to assist with the data analysis. Once transcribed, it is advisable to label the disks then make two back-up 'floppy disk' copies, print one hard copy of the transcript and store these in a separate place. As so many researchers will tell you, the one time when you don't follow this advice will be the transcript you lose.

Another useful pointer, particularly in relation to budgeting or in trying to decide if you will take on the task yourself, concerns the time taken to transcribe tapes. Depending of course on the skill of the transcriber and the clarity of the tape, the following times (Gifford 1992) are an approximate guide:

- 1 hour English interview with 1 person: 3–6 hours;
- 1 hour non-English interview into English: 6–9 hours; and
- 1 hour focus group in English: 6–12 hours

Data processing record

As the volume of my data began to grow, I devised a spread sheet on which I recorded which stages had been completed in the processing of each set of data (Fig. 8.1). The processing stages included on this form were:

- the entry of the session in the data collection log;
- the phases involved with transcribing the audio tapes;

Data processing stages	Groups							
	1	2	3	4	5	6	7	8
Session logged								
Contact summary form completed								
Transcribed								
Checked								
Corrected and converted								
Numbered								
Coded								
Summarised								
Summary and transcript sent								
Comments								

Fig. 8.1 A data processing record

- the conversion, numbering, coding and or other preparation of data for analysis using a computer software package, e.g. Ethnograph (Seidal et al 1988);
- the completion of the analysis summary for return to the participants for validation;
- the completion of the contact summary form; and
- the record of the date the summaries were mailed to the participants.

Data collection log

Although the data collection log was not maintained for the purposes of organising the data, it is described here for the sake of completeness. The log was, in essence, a fieldwork diary. After each contact, interview or workshop, where data for the study was collected, I recorded supplementary information relating to that session. Among the points recorded were:

- the setting and relevant background to the session and/or the individuals providing the information;
- where the session took place;
- the length of the session;
- any prejudgements on my part which I became aware of before, during or after the study;
- my reactions to any aspect of the session or the information it provided; and
- questions that came to mind, or insight gained during or after the session.

The log also provided a written analysis of how the session went, and what changes were indicated for future interviews or workshops. The following log extracts from two of my interviews illustrate several of these points:

#1. 1½ hour interview. The setting of the interview broke just about every rule we are taught in the quantitative paradigm! There were numerous children coming and going during the interview, either demanding their mother's attention or trying to satisfy their curiosity about me. The house was extremely crowded with everything everywhere and we ended up squeezed around the dining room table. At least one phone call interrupted the interview. The scene was obviously the norm, so I guess it added to the authenticity. (In retrospect I'm amazed how congruent the discussion was!)

#2. The courage and balance of these women has to be admired. Being able to survive some of the personal situations and experiences they have been in, and then be able to provide constructive criticism of the system which has so often failed them is almost beyond my understanding. At the end of the interview they turned the tables on me by asking what I had got out of the session. Good example of the sharing approach required in this type of research.

Each session was reflected upon and recorded within two days of its occurrence. This process assisted in identifying possible personal biases that might have distorted the data. In this way the log was one of the strategies employed to enhance the trustworthiness of the data.

Contact summary form

The contact summary form (Fig. 8.2) is designed to sum up the major points that emerge from each data collection session. The headings on this form are specific, being dictated by the particular qualitative methodology being employed, and the research questions being asked. In the case of my study, in which a critical inquiry methodology was used, I wanted to note the themes, issues and contradictions that were emerging from the data. Points that had not arisen in sessions with other groups, which indicated that new information was still being generated (i.e. that data saturation had not yet been reached), and issues that required following up with the participants for clarification or amplification, were also noted on this form.

During the course of my study, the contact summary form served several purposes. Not only did it provide a resume of the material, but it also allowed me to become increasingly familiar with my data. The process of identifying and summarising the themes, issues and contradictions served two additional purposes. It indicated areas where more data were required and also contributed to the analysis. The interweaving of data collection and data analysis illustrated the point that, in the conduct of a qualitative study, there is an absence of the clearly circumscribed stages typical of the quantitative method, and that aspects of the various phases overlap and usually occur concurrently.

Organisation/Group:

Date:

Themes/Issues that emerged
from interview/contact:

Summary of information obtained
on research questions:

Issue   *Information*
Purpose/benefits of community involvement

Problems

Practical forms

Factors affecting implementation
(+ve & -ve)

Means of strengthening/minimising factors

Points to note:

Points to follow up:

Fig. 8.2 A contact summary form

Document record

If you are collecting material from documents, a summary of the data is also
very useful. On the document record form I used for my study, I noted the
organisation to which the document was linked, the number of the document where more than one document per organisation was involved
(referencing details), a summary of content relevant to the research focus,
and an analysis of that content.

Master sheet

A master sheet (Fig. 8.3) may be used to tie all the individual data
generation documents together. This form summarises all the information
recorded on these documents for all respondents in the study. In my study
this master sheet came into being half way through the data collection
process to simplify the keeping-track-of process. Experience has taught me
that this type of document *is necessary* right from the beginning of the study.

Interview	Contact dates	Logged	Contact summary complete	Transcribed	Checked	Corrected and converted	Numbered	Coded	Summary of interview/workshop	Analysis summary/transcript sent	Comments
Executive Officer Health Advisory Network (HAN)	9/6/89	X	N/A	—	—	Not taped	—	—	I	N/A	See also summary Group 1—PHA
Australian Nursing Federation	12/7/89 1 26/6/90 2	X X	X X	X X	X X	X X	X X	X X	1 1	T & S S	
Student Initiatives in Community Health	15/3/90	X	X	Decision not to continue participation in study							
Murray Districts Junior Hospital Board	11/5/90	X	X	—	—	Not taped		—		✓	Advised 18/7 not able to establish Board this year
Public Health Association	2/6/90	X		X	X	X	X	X	W	WS	Policy drafted 10/7
Author–HAN Evaluation Report	19/6/90	X	N/A	—	—	Not taped	—	—	I	N/A	Contextual material

Fig. 8.3 An extract from a master sheet

Filing system

Right from the commencement of your study, you should establish a system whereby you can readily locate a given document. According to Gifford (1992), the components of the basic filing system that needs to be established for a qualitative study are:

- The master file: the original copies of all data including interview scripts, records of observations and the like, field notes, logs;
- The working file: the copies of the contents of the master file which are used as the working copies. The master and the working files should be kept in different locations;
- Theme files: contain material relevant to specific themes or topics identified as the data analysis proceeds. Both data and related memos are included in each file;
- Case files: contain information relating to specific units of analysis, e.g. individuals, communities, organisations. These files may be hard copy and/or on computer disks.

I would reinforce the need to make two copies of all essential material and keep the copies in separate locations.

Analysis

Although, as previously indicated, the analysis phase can not be isolated from other data related processes, there are some components that need to follow the bulk of the data collection, rather than occur concurrently.

Computer software

One common myth which needs to be exploded before proceeding any further, is that relating to the capabilities of computer software packages designed for processing qualitative data, such as Ethnograph mentioned earlier. These packages have been designed to replace the labour intensive cut-and-paste approach to organising data. As such, they do not analyse the data for you. Judging by a number of comments made, both verbally and in research reports, the belief that these packages do just that seems fairly widespread. More sophisticated software, such as 'NUDIST' (Richards & Richards 1991), is available to assist with qualitative data analysis and theory building. Nevertheless, as depressing as the idea may be, these core processes are still a cognitive function required of the researcher. As Michael Agar so succinctly put it, 'you need a lot of right brain' (1991).

The application of computer software to assist in the analysis of qualitative data is a subject on its own and there is not room to address the issues in this chapter. If this is an area with which you are not familiar, I would recommend either *Qualitative research: analysis types and software tools* by Tesch (1990), or *Using computers in qualitative research* by Fielding and Lee (1991). If you are not particularly skilled in computing, attending a course employing one of the software packages described by these writers will usually prove to be worthwhile. Unless you are computer literate, the teach-yourself approach with the aid of an instruction manual can be a very frustrating experience.

Becoming familiar with the data

The first step in the process is to start becoming very conversant with the information you are obtaining. The saying often used in association with qualitative studies of 'living with your data' does, in a sense, reflect the reality. Fortunately, familiarisation is aided by processing the data. I found, for example, that as I checked transcripts against the audiotapes for accuracy to fill in the gaps that my typist had not been able to decipher, and then again to code the transcript, sections of the discussion began to settle in my memory. If you have transcribed the tapes yourself, you become familiar with the content more quickly. This benefit is however offset by the amount of time taken to do the transcribing.

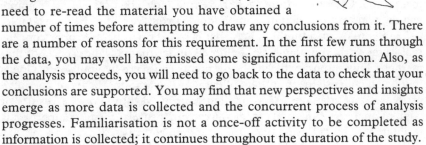

Regardless of who transcribes the tapes, you will need to re-read the material you have obtained a number of times before attempting to draw any conclusions from it. There are a number of reasons for this requirement. In the first few runs through the data, you may well have missed some significant information. Also, as the analysis proceeds, you will need to go back to the data to check that your conclusions are supported. You may find that new perspectives and insights emerge as more data is collected and the concurrent process of analysis progresses. Familiarisation is not a once-off activity to be completed as information is collected; it continues throughout the duration of the study.

Coding

The aim of coding is to identify what various writers have described as themes, patterns, topics or concepts. The process can be undertaken with varying degrees of focus or specificity. As each method of quantitative analysis has its own specific approach to coding, you should check the relevant research texts for the details of the coding format specific to the particular methodology you intend to use.

Recording your progress

Do not rely on your memory for all the insights you gain as you work with the data. These ideas can range from new lines of enquiry to pursue, to alternative interpretations of the data you have been analysing. With all the information you are inputting to your brain, you will be hard pressed to remember these insights as the study progresses. Write down any thoughts you have as soon as possible. A number of terms are used for these notes, for example memos or commentaries.

Progressing the analysis

I found this to be the most difficult stage of the whole process during the conduct of my study. While it was all very well for lecturers and supervisors to trot out phrases like 'live with the data' or 'just cogitate for a while and it will all come together,' I needed something more concrete to go on. Having recognised that I relied on visual cues, I sought out strategies to assist the cognitive process of analysis. For those of you who find auditory input more useful, other strategies can be developed.

Computer software packages such as Ethnograph were a great help at this stage of identifying themes and the like. By being able to pull out all the commonly coded segments from transcripts, my data was consolidated and presented in a manner that provided the visual input I needed to progress with my analysis.

The next step I adopted was to note down all the significant points and themes that I identified from each transcript. How you organise these points will depend on the qualitative methodology you are using. If, for example, you are employing a methodology that is based on a theoretical or conceptual framework, the points can be noted under the relevant aspects of that method. This summary of significant points can serve two purposes. One is that it can collapse the mountain of data into an amount that your cognitive processes can manage. As your data from workshops, or the results of content analysis of documents, are already in a similar form, comparison is facilitated if you are using data from different sources.

Secondly, the material can form a summary of the interview for return to the participants. They can then decide if the summary reflects what they wanted to convey, and if not, what needs to be changed, deleted or added. This contributes to establishing the trustworthiness of the data and hence the validity of the study.

Matrix analysis

Although some reduction in data is achieved by summarising the transcripts, more needs to done. I found entering these significant points on to matrices, a grid-like display of rows, columns and cells, a very useful next step. According to Marsh, (1990):

matrix analysis may be used to help simplify the analysis of qualitative data, condense findings so that they may be more easily communicated, create an audit trail of how credibility was established and obtain confidence in the trustworthiness of findings for both the subjects and the contexts with which qualitative methods are used.

Analysis also is facilitated by the opportunity to visualise large amounts of data simultaneously. For example, the existence of empty cells, or data that fit into more than one category, indicates consideration of redefining categories or providing alternative theoretical explanations.

Miles and Huberman (1984) identified a number of types of matrices classified according to their particular function, e.g. descriptive, process or outcome oriented. The details of these various types can be obtained from that reference. For my study, I developed two types of matrices to facilitate the analysis of my data. As Marsh (1990) advocated, each was 'constructed as a function of (my own) analysis needs and creativity'. (Marsh's article also includes an example of a process oriented matrix which is one of the variety of formats that can be generated.)

The first matrix I devised was exploratory, in that it served to assist in both the exploration of the data that had been generated, and the reduction of that data into more inclusive themes. The second matrix was outcome oriented, being built on the outcomes of the exploratory matrices. The function of this confirmatory matrix was to clarify emerging themes through the process of testing and confirmation. Figures 8.4 and 8.5 are examples of the formats I developed for the exploratory and outcome oriented matrices that I required. Each matrix identified the specific issue being addressed, the objective of the analysis (i.e. exploration or confirmation), and a description of the procedure followed. This latter information allowed for the analytic process used to be easily audited by another researcher. The components of the procedure that are documented here are:

- the particular set of data being analysed;
- the categories of data that are to be entered in the rows and columns of the matrix;
- the decision rules being used to determine the data to be entered;
- the operations to be used in analysing the data entered; and
- the conclusions drawn from this analysis.

What is entered into each matrix cell are condensed segments of data obtained from coded transcripts. Just which bits of data are entered into which cells is determined by the decision rules or criteria established prior to commencing the process. These decision rules must be consistently followed as analysis progresses.

An explanation of the process, using two of the less complex matrices from my research of community participation, may assist in clarifying the procedure.

Research issue: Functions of public involvement
Analysis objective: Exploratory
Description of procedure:

Data set	Matrix	Decision rules	Analysis operations	Conclusions drawn
Summaries of significant statements from coded transcripts	*Rows:* Participant groups *Columns:* Four themes identified from reading of several summaries: • advisory • advocacy • communication channel • assistance with activities	Data to be entered: • List words/phrases relevant to the four themes in column 2. • Add new themes to matrix as/if they emerge	Review matrix for additional or alternative themes, areas of overlap, etc. Identify over-arching categories and sub-categories	Two major functions: (a) Ideal: • empowerment (b) Instrumental: • communication • provision of care • management

Fig. 8.4 An exploratory matrix

Research issue: Functions of public involvement
Analysis objective: Clarification of emerging themes (testing and confirmation)
Description of procedure:

Data set	Matrix	Decision rules	Analysis operations	Conclusions drawn
Exploratory matrix for 'Functions of Community Involvement'.	Two matrices: (a) *Ideal:* Rows = participant groups Column = empowerment (b) *Instrumental:* Three columns: • communication • provision of care • management.	Data to be entered: (a) *Empowerment:* Words/phrases relating to the concept at the individual or community level, e.g. political pressure, advocacy, self-help (in general terms) (b) *Words/phrases relating to the three instrumental themes.*	Comparison across participant group Review content of matrix cells	Identified themes supported by content of matrices (no major gaps) and data supplied by participants covered by the themes. Matrices do not indicate that the data can be reduced any further

Fig. 8.5 A confirmatory matrix

Exploratory matrices. An exploratory matrix was constructed for each aspect or issue raised by the study participants. The data sets used as a basis for these matrices were the summaries I had made of significant themes identified in the coded transcripts. The participating groups formed the rows of the matrices, and the themes which had been identified from the summaries as being relevant to the particular issue being explored, formed the columns. Taking the issue of functions of public involvement as an example (Fig. 8.6), the provisional themes heading the columns in this exploratory matrix were 'Advisory, Advocacy, Communication Channel and Assistance with Activities.' Using the significant statements that had been extracted from the transcripts as the source, the words or phrases related to these four themes were entered into the cells. As this progressed, the comparison between the data that been entered into cells, and the data in the source documents which did not fit with the provisional categories indicated that additional categories needed to be generated. In the case of this particular matrix, no additional categories were needed.

I found that this stage needed to be done manually, as large sheets of paper (or alternatively tiny writing!) were required to visualise the total matrix. Don't be fooled by the neat matrix presented in Figure 8.6. Like that of my colleagues, my first draft of the matrix was far from being this organised—with data that did not clearly fit into any of the existing categories being entered across two adjacent columns, and notes or questions jotted here and there.

Once all the information has been entered, the matrix can be reviewed for categories that are not supported by substantial data (i.e. a number of empty cells in the column), categories that are confirmed and any areas of overlap. Categories can then be collapsed and data combined. Where only a few cells contain data, the related category should be dropped as there is no evidence of a common theme. In some cases, however, it may be feasible to transfer the data in these cells to a related category. Throughout the process of comparison you must, as Marsh emphasised, 'remain open to discovering similarities, differences and emerging patterns in the data' (1990).

The outcome of this process is the identification of overreaching categories that encompass a number of sub categories. In the example provided, the conclusions drawn at the end of this analytic process were that there were two major functions of public involvement identified by the participants: ideal and instrumental. The ideal function related to the empowerment of the community while the instrumental functions related to communication, provision of care and management of services.

Confirmatory matrices. The framework for the next set of matrices devised for my study were the conclusions drawn from exploratory matrices. As the name suggests, the confirmatory matrices had as their objective the clarification, testing and confirmation of these emerging themes. Once again the participant groups formed the rows of the matrices while the overreaching categories identified from the exploratory matrices constituted the columns.

PARTICIPANTS	THEMES			
	Advisory	Advocacy	Communication channel	Assistance with activities
South East Community Development Council	Identification of needs Source of new ideas Policy, planning Service overlap	Control vested in community Empowerment community and individual	Linking resources	'Hands-on' co-ordination, liaison, facilitating training • limits to degree/types • ethical considerations • legal requirements
Carers' Forum	Problems Practicalities Alternative perspectives, approaches	Empowerment of individuals Advocacy for members Stimulant to system (complacency)	Linking people and services Information Between members	Volunteers
N. Hospital Board	Input on community needs Management control— joint responsibility	Political pressure Empowerment of individuals	Channel between service managers and public; e.g. needs, concerns, explanations	Volunteers—use of community expertise Co-ordination Educational purposes Services—extras (govt—basics)

Fig. 8.6 Example of an extract from an exploratory matrix: functions of public involvement

THEMES

PARTICIPANTS	Communication	Provision of care	Management
Youth Health	Information Linkage between groups (community health care professionals, management).	Self-help groups—support. Volunteers. Areas not covered (e.g. education, resources).	Feedback to providers. Realistic limits required.
Australian Nursing Federation	More than consultation. Information Advisory—identification of: needs, differences new ways of meeting needs.	Self-help care.	Face-to-face feedback more effective. More efficient health care through increased personal and community responsibility. Broadens horizons—change in approach to services delivery.
Royal College of Nursing, Australia	Dissemination of information, increased awareness of resources. Consult/canvass community opinion. Advisory—needs, resources, policy formulation.	Self-help groups/networks	Delegate small areas. Stimulate change.

Fig. 8.7 Example of an extract from a confirmatory matrix: instrumental functions of community involvement

Taking the instrumental functions of public involvement (Fig. 8.7) as an example from my study, the themes heading the matrix columns were 'Communication, Provision of Care and Management.' The names of the specific participant groups were entered into the rows. Working from the related exploratory matrix, words or phrases associated with these themes were entered into the appropriate cells. Once this entry process was completed, it was possible to determine whether the identified themes were supported by the data, i.e. that there were no empty cells, and that all the data supplied by the participant groups had found a home in one of the cells. Consideration was also given as to whether any of the themes that had been identified could be further reduced through combination. As all these criteria were met. then the themes that had been identified were considered to have been confirmed.

Conclusion

By now you may have come to the conclusion that this seeming plethora of documents may be more of a hindrance than a help. While this may be the case for you, for others it will not be so. What you need to decide is what works best for you in terms of organising and monitoring the data you are generating. In my case, the documents described here provided me with a sense of being in control of the process—indeed a sense of security that was very comforting at various stages of a long process which stretched from my original idea to my finished report.

REFERENCES

Agar M 1991 The right brain strikes back. In: Fielding M, Lee R (eds) Using computers in qualitative research. Sage, London, p 194

Fielding N, Lee R 1991 Using computers in qualitative research. Sage, London

Gifford S 1992 Course materials for the short course on qualitative methods in health science research. Department of Social and Preventative Medicine, Monash University, Melbourne

Marsh G 1990 Refining an emergent lifestyle: change theory through matrix analysis. Advances in Nursing Science 12(3):41–52

Miles M, Huberman A 1984 Qualitative data analysis. Sage, Beverley Hills

Seidal J, Kjolseth R, Seymour E 1988 Ethnograph: a user's guide, version 3.0. Qualis, Littleton, Colorado

Tesch R 1990 Qualitative research analysis and software tools. Falmer, London

Walker B 1993 Computer analysis of qualitative data: a comparison of three packages. Qualitative Health Research 3(1):91–111

Watts R 1992 Rhetoric or reality: a critical analysis of public involvement in the Western Australian health care system. Unpublished PhD thesis, University of Colorado, Denver

9. Disseminating findings

Jeanette Robertson

Writing for publication

Apart from the personal recognition and enhanced opportunities for promotion that may occur following the publication of an article, nurses need access to research findings in order to incorporate new knowledge into their practice and improve patient care. As a natural conclusion to the research process, therefore, the findings of any valid and reliable project should be 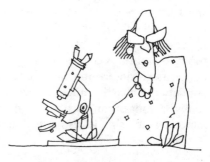 prepared for submission to an appropriate journal. In addition to reporting research findings, articles which describe legal, ethical, methodological and practical aspects of undertaking research should also be written up for publication. These articles are often favourably regarded by those journal editors keen to expose the process as well as the outcomes of research to their readers.

Regardless of the subject however, student assignments submitted to journals in their original form are seldom considered suitable for publication. This is because their content, length and organisation are usually very different from the type of copy sought after by journal editors, and for this reason the rejection of course work submitted in its original form can almost be guaranteed. If reworked, however, most reports, theses and assignments do have the potential to become journal articles. If you are contemplating publishing course work, you should refer to the specialised texts (referenced at the end of this chapter) which deal with the transformation of student assignments into journal articles.

Before beginning to write up the findings of your research into a publishable format, you should decide upon your target audience and consider the most appropriate journal in which to publish your findings. The determination of these objectives may facilitate the preparation of your article, as you can write with the (perceived) needs of a specific group of readers in mind.

The selection of a suitable journal is vital to the process of information dissemination and must be undertaken with extreme care. This is because articles published in inappropriate journals are less likely to reach to their target readership than are those which appear in journals selected on the basis of their relevance to the article and its purpose.

Choosing a journal

Currently there are some seventy nursing journals which contribute to nursing knowledge and improve the delivery of nursing care. As each of these journals aims to fill a specific gap in the nursing literature, there are many titles from which to choose. Your first step therefore is to compile a short list of potentially suitable journals. To do this, refer to the subject headings classification in the journal indexes (e.g. CINAHL, *International Nursing Index*), and note those titles which publish articles relevant to your topic. Obtain a recent edition of each of these journals and examine the contents to determine the scope, complexity, and style of the articles contained. Once this initial review has been undertaken, you should be able to revise your original list and consider the time, geographical and prestige factors, which should also influence your choice of journal.

Potential readership

The most important question to ask yourself when contemplating writing for publication is 'who do I want to read the article?' Generally speaking, if your article is relevant to all aspects of nursing practice, then publication in a general nursing journal should be considered. Articles which address highly specialised aspects of nursing care, however, are best submitted to publications which deal with the relevant nursing specialty.

Style and emphasis

Whether generalised or focused on a specialised branch of practice, every nursing journal aims to maintain consistency in the style of articles it publishes. As there is considerable variety between journals, you should select one which contains articles congruent with the scope and complexity of your own.

Place of publication

If the content of your article is specific to a particular area, state or country, then publication in a journal which serves the population encompassed by the subject matter is usually your only option. If the content is universally relevant, however, your choice increases significantly as publishing in overseas journals becomes an additional option.

The benefits of publishing overseas include a wider choice of titles and a wider readership. On the debit side, however, are the long time delays which are often incurred between the submission and publication of your article, and the need to modify both your style and spelling to conform with the usage of the country where the journal is published. These modifications are particularly necessary when writing for American journals where differences in spelling are commonly encountered.

Frequency of publication

Journals which are published monthly have a far quicker turnover of material, and a shorter time lag between submission and review, than those which are published bi-monthly or quarterly. For this reason, articles which contain information with the potential to date should be offered to journals which are published at least bi-monthly.

Refereed and non-refereed journals

Generally speaking publications appearing in refereed journals carry more prestige than those appearing in their non-refereed counterparts. For this reason, if personal recognition is a primary motivation to publish, you should submit your article to a refereed journal, as it is these publications which have the potential to confer significant prestige upon authors for their contribution to nursing practice.

If your desire to publish outweighs the prospect of rejection, you may prefer to submit your article to a non-refereed journal, where it may be more easily accepted. Notwithstanding this motivation however, the circumstances surrounding the origin of your paper may also dictate whether or not it needs to be subjected to the scrutiny of referees. For example, if the article deals with contemporary issues, not amenable to the time lags encountered while the (often lengthy) review process is in progress, publication in a non-refereed journal is almost certainly your preferred option.

After considering all these factors you should now be in a position to decide where you should submit your article. When you have made this decision, obtain a copy of a recent edition of your chosen journal and read the style guide carefully.

Style guides

Style guides are essential reading for anyone contemplating submitting an article for publication. Usually found under the heading 'advice to contributors', style guides normally stipulate:

- the journal's preferred subject areas;
- the length and format of articles;

- the requirements for the presentation of any figures, tables, illustrations or photographs;
- accepted reference styles;
- the time frame for publication; and
- contact addresses.

The directions contained in style guides should be followed to the letter when preparing your manuscript, as in most cases articles will not be considered for publication unless they conform to the format specified in the journal's style guide.

Format of a research article

Having decided upon your target audience and journal, you are now ready to begin writing your article. Traditionally articles reporting research findings have adhered to the format described by Tornquist (1986), viz. an introduction, a statement of the research question, a description of the research methodology and results, and the discussion and recommendations.

Introduction

The purpose of the introduction is to attract the reader's interest by placing the nursing problem which motivated your study into its context. In your opening paragraphs include the reasons for undertaking the research and a brief review of the literature, which either describes the significant findings of any similar studies already completed or justifies the extension of another study. If there is an identifiable deficit in the literature, this should also be reported, as a lack of information about a nursing problem is, in itself, a reason for undertaking research. Once you have completed the literature review, conclude the introduction with a brief statement as to the purpose of your research and the possible implications of your study.

Stating the research question or hypothesis

The definition of the research question or hypothesis should serve as a logical extension of the introduction. Although no new evidence to support the need for the study should be introduced at this point, a brief statement which summarises the relevant literature can serve as a useful introduction to your definition of the research question or hypothesis.

The research problem is normally expressed as a formal question using either the present or future tense, e.g. will the incidence of colonisation of burn wounds by respiratory pathogens increase if masks are not worn while redressing these wounds?

This is in contrast to a hypothesis statement which can be informally expressed as an expectation which demonstrates a link between two variables, e.g. there will be no difference in the colonisation of burn wounds by respiratory pathogens if masks are not worn when redressing these wounds.

Describing the research methodology

In this section you must describe the methods used in your study in enough detail to allow readers not only to assess the relevance of the findings to their own practice, but also to allow them to replicate the study in their own setting should they wish to do so. In aiming to satisfy these basic requirements, you should begin your description of the research methodology with a statement about the setting of the study and the study population.

The setting. Begin with a general statement which describes the type of health care agency used in the study, e.g. 250 bed paediatric hospital, remote community nursing post, 10 bed same day surgical unit, and briefly outline those aspects of the agency which were relevant to the variables investigated in the study, e.g. casemix, patient facilities. If you had a choice between several similar venues, mention the factors which influenced your decision to undertake the research in your chosen setting.

The sample. In this section describe who and how many subjects comprised your sample, the criteria for their inclusion (or exclusion) in the study population and the methods you used to select the participants. The process used to allocate the study subjects to any groups called for by the methodology should also be described here.

Intervention. If a change to traditional practice constituted the basis of your study, give an account of both the old and new procedures and describe how you went about implementing the change to practice. Include a definition of any unfamiliar or vague terms included in the description (e.g. toddler, fever), so as to leave no doubt about how these terms were interpreted in your study.

Although this description should be relatively brief, it should include enough detail to allow readers to assess the relevance of the intervention to the research question—and the feasibility of implementing a similar change in another setting.

Data collection. The purpose of this section is to allow your readers to evaluate the suitability of the data collection instruments you used. Begin by identifying the variables or interventions measured in the study and describe the methods you employed to collect your data. If you used more than one type of instrument to collect your data, include a brief overview of each type of tool before describing each one individually—moving from the most sensitive, e.g. measures of physiological function, to the less precise, general instruments, e.g. the broad based questionnaire.

Where precise measures were used to collect the data, describe their function and justify their use in terms of their validity. If more than one instrument was used, include a statement as to how you calibrated the instruments to ensure the reliability of the data. If you used a questionnaire, describe the range of topics you covered, and to illustrate the depth and breadth of your survey, include a few carefully chosen examples of relevant questions. If your data collection instrument is well known, do not spend time describing it at length. Instead, outline any modifications you made to the tool and how you established its validity and reliability before administering it to the study sample. If you used medical records to gather data, list the type of information you obtained from this source, e.g. diagnosis, length of stay, drug therapy, etc.

As well as describing the tools, include a description of the data collection process and the measures you took to protect the rights of the participants.

Information which reports successful strategies used to recruit, test, or administer questionnaires is often very useful to new researchers, and therefore a brief report of the practical aspects of the data collection process is usually appreciated by readers embarking on studies utilising a similar design.

Reporting your results

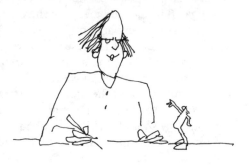

Before presenting your findings, briefly recall the purpose of the study and the composition of the study population. An explanation of any factors which contributed to any discrepancies between the characteristics of the population sample defined in the original research proposal and that used in the study should also be included, as should the rate of attrition and the factors which contributed to the loss of these subjects.

Begin reporting your results by describing the outcome of your study in general terms. If the study incorporated a change in practice, report the results of pre- and post-tests and describe the differences between the findings, initially without referring to any statistical analysis you may have undertaken. Similarly, if experimental and control groups were used, outline the differences and similarities in the results obtained.

If there was no intervention, report on the most important findings of the study first, before moving on to the less crucial (although sometimes more interesting) results. Report only those findings which have relevance to the study question, rather than all of the data generated by the study. Condense your information as much as possible using concise descriptions and figures or tables to represent the important aspects of your work. Keep in mind however that tables are expensive to typeset and take up considerable space, and for this reason, articles containing many tables are not always favoured by editors with tight budgets and space restrictions. You should therefore reserve your tables for the representation of crucial data sets, which cannot be easily described.

After presenting an overview of your results, relate the findings back to the research question or hypothesis. If there are unexpected results, include an explanation of the factors which may have contributed to the outcome. At this point include any statistical analyses you undertook to test the significance of your results. Be sure that the tests you describe are suited to the task however—as statistics which are used or reported inappropriately can detract from the credibility of an otherwise valuable study.

Discussion

The object of the discussion section is to highlight the important findings of your study, outline its limitations, make recommendation for further research and describe how your results can be used to improve patient care. In discussing your findings, compare your results with those of other similar studies and comment on those factors which may have contributed to any discrepancies between your findings and those of other researchers.

Any factors which may have limited the scope of your study should be mentioned here as these can affect the validity, reliability, generalisability or usefulness of the findings. You should also mention any aspects of the data collection process (e.g. problems with the study sample or the setting) which may have influenced the outcome of the study.

Anecdotal notes or findings which emerged by chance (serendipitous findings) can also be included in this section, together with suggestions for further research which will address the limitations identified in your study.

To conclude your discussion, describe how the findings of your research can be used to improve patient care (in spite of its limitations). Use the information derived from your results to make your recommendations as practical statements which suggest strategies that can reasonably be expected to be implemented in the setting where the research was undertaken.

The final paragraph of your article should clearly summarise the focus of the research and the implications of the results. Use catchy words and innuendo if you must—but don't confuse your readers by being too obtuse. It may be the downfall of an otherwise excellent paper.

Acknowledgments

Acknowledgments are a useful means by which to thank those people who have assisted you in your study. If you plan to identify individuals, obtain their permission to do so, and allow them to read your article upon request—to confirm their desire to be associated with your research. If you include names, be certain to spell them correctly.

Abstract

Once you have completed your article, briefly summarise the purpose of the study, the methods used and the findings to compile an abstract. The required length of an abstract varies between journals, and often a great deal of skill is required to condense its contents into a paragraph which accurately represents your research. Even when words are limited, always include a statement as to the reason for undertaking the study and the problem studied. The characteristics of the sample and the setting are also important components of an abstract—as is a statement about the type of methodology used and a summary of the results. Your finished product should contain sufficient information to allow readers to ascertain the relevance of your work to their practice without needing access to the entire article.

Title

Whilst a catchy title (e.g. 'Stop laughing, this is serious') might allow insight into your creative imagination, if it does not relate directly to the subject matter of your article, (e.g. undertaking research using children as subjects), it will be exceedingly difficult to trace during a literature search. You must therefore give your article a title which will allow both librarians and/or your readers to find it easily. If you can incorporate one of the National Library of Medicine Medical Subject Headings (MeSH) into the title this will certainly facilitate the search process; however if this is not possible, ensure that you use one of these 'keywords' in the abstract.

With a title and an abstract, your draft is ready for its first critique and should be given to a colleague to read. Although this person should be conversant with the subject area of the study, it is often preferable to choose someone who knows little about the research process. This is because aspects of the methodology which are not clearly described, or flaws in the logical development of your ideas, will be easily identified by someone who cannot read in the missing words or steps, or comprehend your use of language. Use your reviewer's comments to make minor amendments to your text, but do not make any major changes without seeking a second opinion.

After your draft has been completed, you should re-read your style guide to ensure that you have satisfied all the criteria for submission. In addition to the specific requirements, you should note that all journal editors expect copy to be typed on one side of the paper and to be double spaced. As wide margins facilitate the review and composition process, you should allow at least a 2.5 cm margin around the text on each page. It is also a universal requirement of editors that articles be free of typographical and grammatical errors, jargon, unqualified abbreviations and spelling mistakes. If using a word processor to prepare your article, use the spell and grammar check facilities to identify and correct mistakes. Your final copy should also reflect the spelling and usage of the country where your article is to be submitted (e.g. pediatric vs paediatric, colonise vs colonize, nappy vs diaper).

Once you are satisfied with the final draft, ask a colleague to read it—to confirm the clarity of content and to detect any grammatical, typographical and spelling errors you may have overlooked. It is only when the corrections which arise from this final review have been made that your article is ready for submission.

Enquiry letters

To assist in the planning of individual issues of a journal, some editors request writers to either advise them of the subject or provide an abstract of their article prior to submitting it for consideration. Although this requirement varies between journals, an enquiry letter to the editor is generally a good idea if you are uncertain as to the suitability of the topic or focus of your article for any journal.

Submitting your article

Once confirmation of interest has been received and proof reading has been completed, prepare your article for posting. The journal's style guide will advise you as to the format and number of copies required by the editor, and you should make this number and then one more for yourself as insurance against loss or damage in transit. Ensure that each copy is complete and fastened together with a paper clip (rather than a staple which may damage the pages during its subsequent removal).

Enclose a covering letter with your article which briefly describes the origin of your study and your reasons for selecting the chosen journal. Include details of your qualifications and current position, and to facilitate future contact, your address, telephone number, and if you have one, your fax number.

Wrap your copy securely in a heavy duty envelope and attach stamps which will cover the cost of first class postage. Although often expensive, it is imperative that you use airmail if posting your article overseas, as sea mail or even surface air lifted (SAL) mail often takes months to reach its destination, thereby adding further to the publication lag time.

Journal editors will normally acknowledge the receipt of all manuscripts and you should therefore expect to receive confirmation of arrival within six weeks of posting. Unless your article is obviously unsuitable for the journal, (e.g. by virtue of its subject matter) the acknowledgment will make no reference as to its prospects for publication, and it is not until the review process has been completed that you can expect to hear from the editor again.

If you have not received notification of the safe arrival of your manuscript three months after posting, write to the editor requesting information as to its status. If the reply indicates the article never reached its destination, then you will need to repeat the process of posting the article (using the copy you retained for such catastrophes as a master). Occasionally it is the editor's reply that becomes lost in the mail, and this is easily remedied by the journal staff, either with a copy of the original acknowledgment or a letter advising you of the progress of the review process.

Review process

For non-refereed journals, review of articles are normally undertaken by the editor. For referred publications, however, usually two or three members of the journal's editorial board who have the relevant subject expertise participate in the review process. To eliminate the possibility of any bias towards known authors, reviewers are blinded to the writer's identity when assessing manuscripts.

In addition to the requirements for authors to adhere to the specifications of the style guide and to the laws of spelling and grammar, reviewers expect articles to demonstrate:

- concise, logical development of ideas;
- sound argument and defence of original ideas;
- accuracy of content;
- adequate documentation;
- sound research methodology; and
- congruity with the purpose of the journal (*Nursing Administration Quarterly* in Sheridan & Dowdney, 1986).

It is on the basis of these criteria that your article will be assessed by the reviewers. Four to six months is not an uncommon time for review, so don't get too agitated if you don't hear about the fate of your article before this. It is only after reading the reviewer's reports the editor will be able to make a decision as to the fate of your article and advise you accordingly. Although there are three options open to editors, in practice only two of them, viz. accept with modification or reject, are regularly used. The third—accept as submitted—is a rare event happening to only 5% of the manuscripts submitted to good journals (Day, 1989).

Accept but modify letters

If your article has satisfied the reviewers, you can expect to receive a letter which indicates your hard work has been 'accepted pending modifications.' This type of letter is normally accompanied by the comments of the reviewers and your manuscript which may look somewhat different from the pristine condition in which it left you some months earlier.

Rather than bemoan the heavy use of the reviewers pencil which you may well find rampant throughout your manuscript, read the comments carefully. You will normally find them constructive and extremely helpful in modifying your copy. While it should be said that you do not necessarily have to make any of the minor changes suggested by the reviewers, if the same comment is made by more than one person, it would be wise to do so before returning your article. If you do decide to revise your copy, be sure to meet any deadline stipulated by the editor, as offers to publish articles following modification will normally lapse if the revised manuscript is not received by the date specified.

If a major revision is requested by the editor, take a moment to consider whether the amount of rewriting requested is justified in terms of the effect major modifications will have on the original purpose of the article. If you feel the editor may have misinterpreted the purpose of your work, it may be as well to try another journal rather than lose the original idea through an extensive rewrite. The choice to rewrite the article or try another journal is, however, ultimately yours.

Reject letters

As approximately 50% of all manuscripts are rejected by editorial boards, do not be too disappointed if the editor of your chosen journal finds your article 'not suitable for inclusion.' Usually the reason for rejection will fall into one of three categories.

Sometimes editors unconditionally reject an article because it fails to comply with their journal's requirements with regard to clarity of content or any one of the other criteria previously listed. Although many journals will send a detailed letter which explains the reasons for rejection, others will merely send an impersonal rejection slip, which is of little help to you when reconsidering the fate of your article. Fortunately this type of rejection is uncommon and often arises when writers submit their work to inappropriate journals or fail to fulfil the journal requirements as stipulated in the respective style guides.

The second type of rejection may recognise the merit of your idea, but may justify rejection of the article on the basis of inadequate data or the means you used to collect or process it. Alternatively, the letter may identify parts of the manuscript which could be improved with extensive revision of the text, the collection of more data and/or the revision of your results so that they reflect the available evidence. It is important to realise that this type of rejection differs from the 'accept after modification' letter as there is no commitment from the editor to publish, even after an extensive rewrite which takes into account all the reviewer's comments. It is merely an indication of how you might improve your chances of having your article published, but without any promises attached. On this basis, you may be wise to try another journal with your improved copy.

The third kind of rejection is the most promising for authors as it usually identifies one major defect, which is normally easily rectified. Almost as good as the accept with modifications letter, articles which are returned with this reject notice should be revised to include the information requested and returned to the same journal as quickly as possible—together with a covering letter which describes the new material included in the revised edition of the article.

Proof reading

After your article has been accepted, and before publication, most journal editors will expect you to check the galley proofs to detect typesetting errors and confirm the sense of the text. When proof reading, carefully examine every word individually as well as in its context as the transposed letter (e.g. sing here as opposed to sign here) will be as misleading to the reader as letters which are omitted (e.g. sin here), added (e.g. sign there) or substituted (e.g. sigh here). To facilitate the review process, Day (1989) advocates reading the text aloud to identify the errors inadvertently made by typesetters not familiar with nursing language, your name, or the names of those whom you may have mentioned in the acknowledgments.

If you have incorporated tables in your article, scrutinise every number in every table to ensure that what is printed is an accurate representation of your results. Check the labelling of the axes of any graphs you may have included and also that any photographs or other illustrations are the right way up. (To facilitate this process mark 'TOP' on the back of each illustration you submit with your article.)

Correct any mistakes in accordance with the instructions supplied with the proofs. At this late stage you should not be adding any new material to the article as it invariably causes problems for the publisher. If you detect the omission of lines or words from the original text however, by all means make the necessary corrections. When you have thoroughly checked your proofs, return them to the publisher by the date stipulated via first class mail.

By now all there is to do is wait for the release of the designated issue of 'your' journal. The personal satisfaction which you will almost certainly experience when you finally see your hard work in print is worth the all the hard work you put into developing your article, all the anxiety you may have experienced whilst awaiting the outcome of the review process and the disappointment you probably felt when reading the (sometimes blunt) criticism levelled at your work by faceless referees. While these burdens may have been hard to endure at the time, all will pale into insignificance when your article is published in the journal of your choice.

Oral presentations at seminars and conferences

While the publication of research findings ultimately has the potential to reach a wider audience, the opportunity to speak at a conference will allow you to present your findings relatively soon after completing your study. In addition, as oral presentations are not subject to the constraints imposed by the formal journal style guides, you will be able to incorporate the elements of flair and creativity not always sought after by journal editors.

Once you receive notification that your abstract has been accepted, it is perfectly normal to feel apprehensive at the thought of condensing many months work into some ten or fifteen minutes. It is in fact a positive sign as, providing you can control your nerves, the extra adrenaline should contribute to a lively delivery of your paper and enhance your credibility as a valuable contributor to nursing knowledge. In every oral presentation, the key to a competent and enjoyable talk is careful preparation and rehearsal of the content.

Preparing the content

Giving a talk is much more than reading an article prepared for publication. This is because the detailed descriptions of the research process, often sought after by journal editors, are difficult to comprehend during an oral presentation. Bearing this in mind, your audience is far more likely to appreciate the value of your project if you provide them with a concise overview of your methodology and focus the bulk of the presentation on the implications of your most important findings. To this end when preparing your talk, you should consider dividing the content into three distinct parts, viz. the introduction, the main body and the conclusion.

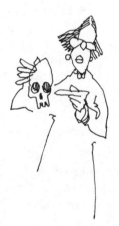

Introduction

The purpose of the introduction is to get the attention of the audience so that you can deliver your message. To attract attention, Grimmond (1992) recommends you use a relevant controversial statement, interesting statistic, or pertinent anecdotal story to set your research in context. Once you have the audience listening, plan to relate the circumstances which gave rise to your study and to give an overview of the literature which describes the findings of any previous research undertaken on the same or a similar problem. Your introduction should conclude with a statement of your research question/hypothesis, and what you hoped to achieve by undertaking the research.

Body of the talk

The main body of your talk should briefly outline the research methodology and your most important findings. Include a description of the subjects included in (and excluded from) your study, the setting where you undertook the research, and the methods you employed to collect your data. As some of your audience will not be familiar with your chosen subject area, you should also include a definition of any unusual or crucial terms you plan to use during the talk. This part of your talk should conclude with the presentation of your results. Plan to present only your most important findings as simply as possible, using appropriate visual aids to give emphasis to the major points (five major points is plenty), which will leave your audience in no doubt as to the outcome of your study.

Conclusion

The conclusion should summarise your results, and relate them back to the research question and the original reason for undertaking the study. Once you have answered your research question in the light of the findings, you may like to speculate on the usefulness of the results for nursing practice in your area, and for nursing in general. In the light of any limitations of your methodology encountered during the conduct of your study, your closing statement may make recommendations for further studies which replicate or extend your study.

Formatting your notes

Once you have drafted your content, have it typed in large letters on numbered pages with a margin wide enough to write in your cues for your visual aids or other prompts. Highlight the main points in the text so that they are easily recognisable at a glance.

Preparation of visual aids

Overhead projection films

Overhead films are an easy-to-prepare, economical way of presenting visual material. They can be prepared before your talk and are particularly useful in rooms where the light cannot be totally eliminated, or where light is needed during the presentation. Overheads also have the advantage of allowing you to reveal your information progressively, or build on a concept using overlays.

When preparing overheads, use the portrait, or vertical, orientation. Otherwise, unless the projector's stage is wide enough to take landscape views, you will need to move your films sideways during the presentation. Avoid crowding your information, and limit the content of each sheet to approximately seven lines of text by using simple phrases to express your key points. Where possible use computer graphics and laser printers to produce your text in 30 point upper and lower case letters. While the Helvetica or Times fonts are easiest to read, any font (other than a cursive script) will suffice.

If handwriting your overheads, ensure each letter is at least eight millimetres in height. If you use coloured pens, limit your selection to two or three shades. As yellow and orange tones become almost invisible when projected, they should be avoided.

Never contemplate screening sheets of typewritten text or text photo-copied from a book. The type face is invariably too small to be deciphered, and the quality of the film is usually very poor. If you wish to use diagrams from a published source, enlarge them to the size of an A4 sheet and try them out during rehearsal to assess their clarity.

Slides

The use of relevant, attractive slides can save you many words and therefore precious minutes during your presentation. As slides allow concepts which are difficult to describe to be meaningfully presented, they can be an invaluable adjunct to your talk. If poorly prepared or presented, however, they can equally spoil your presentation.

When preparing text for slides you should follow the guidelines for preparing overhead films, but limit the text to six words to a line and six lines to a slide. When taking photographs to present with your talk, eliminate all content not relevant to the point of the slide in the picture and ensure that the background is uncluttered as possible.

Rehearsing your talk

Rehearsals are a particularly important phase of your preparation as they enable you to tailor your content to the time available, and to identify and revamp those parts of your paper which are difficult to deliver—before you present your talk. During the early rehearsals, it is not necessary to verbalise the contents of your paper. Silently reading the text will suffice until you are fully conversant with the format of the material. As the date of your presentation approaches, however, you should practise manipulating your visual aids in conjunction with a verbal rehearsal of your paper. At this stage, it may be helpful to invite an objective observer to listen to your talk and check your slides or overheads for clarity. If this opportunity is not available, tape your talk and listen to the recording to ensure that your main points are clearly stated, and that the content moves in a logical sequence from beginning to end.

With a comprehensive preparation, the chances of leaving a good impression on your audience are increased. There are however aspects of presenting a paper which can increase the quality of your presentation even further.

Presenting your talk

The first rule when presenting a paper is 'know how the audio visual aids work before you start to speak.' Use the conference sessions before you to observe how other speakers manage the venue and equipment. Use the breaks between sessions to practise operating the equipment. During practice, project your slides or overhead films onto the screen to check that they are in the correct order, in focus and the right way up. If using overhead transparencies, negotiate with the chairperson of your session as to who will change the overheads, and decide upon a suitable cue to indicate when you wish to have the film changed. If you have not already done so, number your slides and films sequentially to preserve their order, and mark your slides to indicate their orientation in the carousel or cartridge.

If, after your introduction you start with a joke, make it a very good one. If you can't be funny, don't try, as the audience will invariably be put off the rest of your performance by an unfavourable beginning. Once into your presentation, use the confidence gained during rehearsals to speak to your paper, rather than read it verbatim. Use your notes to ensure that you have covered all your main points, and your slides as cues to move from point to point. If possible relate your material to the experience of the audience as this will establish a link between your study and their practice setting and make your presentation more meaningful to them. Where possible use appropriate anecdotal experiences to illustrate your points but avoid poor humour, complex language or in house jargon, which are likely to distract, embarrass or (worse still) alienate your audience.

Move your eyes around the room as you speak to give the audience the impression that you are really speaking to them—rather than the clock on the wall. If you have rehearsed your content thoroughly, this should be relatively easy to achieve, and you should only need to refer to your notes to cue in your slides and check to see that you have covered all your material.

When presenting your slides or overhead films, face the audience rather than the screen. Rather than reading the text verbatim simply explain what the slide is about and then wait a moment to allow the audience to absorb the information in front of them. Before moving on, re-emphasise the main points of your text, as concurrent visual and verbal information is more likely to be retained than either form of input presented in isolation. If you have a long break between slides, use a blank slide rather than leaving an old concept on the screen. Similarly, if the next overhead film is not immediately required turn off the overhead projector.

A single statement, which reflects the purpose of the study, and leaves the audience with a final message regarding future practice, is a useful way to finish your presentation. You may also like to thank your audience before leaving the podium or taking questions. On no account use the term 'in conclusion' unless you mean to finish, as you will more than likely immediately lose the attention of your audience.

Taking questions

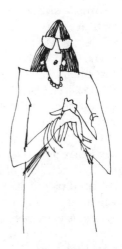

Questions are an important part of any presentation as they allow the audience to seek clarification or request extra information on some aspect of your paper. When taking questions, listen carefully and request that the question be repeated if you can't hear or don't understand what is being asked. Paraphrase the question for the audience if necessary and keep your replies brief and to the point. If you don't know the answer, have the courage to say so, as attempts to bluff your way through will invariably lead you into trouble. Where feasible, offer to contact the person when you have the information, but don't make promises you can't (or don't intend to) keep.

If you cannot reasonably reply to a question without going into a lengthy explanation, give a brief overview of the main issues and invite the person who asked the question to consult you during the break for a detailed reply. Reserve this strategy for only the most complex queries, as people will be deterred from participating in this important phase of your presentation if you continually evade answering their questions.

Despite the butterflies that accompany the experience, presenting the findings of you research at a conference can be a very rewarding experience. Public speaking is not everyone's forte, however, and there is another way if you feel that you simply cannot face an audience.

Presenting your research findings as a poster

With the upsurge in the nursing research, the poster has emerged as an valuable method of presenting research findings. Although possibly not (yet) carrying the prestige of an oral presentation, poster sessions are becoming increasingly popular at nursing conferences. This is because there is the potential for a greater degree of interaction between the researcher and consumers of research. As the presenter of the poster is normally available to answer questions, there is a far greater opportunity to probe aspects of the study in greater detail than is possible following an oral presentation.

Types of posters

The most successful posters are those which are not only carefully designed to attract an audience but also which present research findings accurately and concisely. There are a number of different ways to present a poster, and in the main your choice will be governed by the limitations of the display setting and the distance you will need to transport your poster.

Single sheet. Traditionally posters have been mounted on a single sheet of heavy duty card. For a poster which is to be presented nearby, this form of display is still perfectly acceptable—particularly if mounted on poster board and/or backed with a slab of polystyrene foam or similar reinforcement which makes it less likely to curl at the edges. Although popular for local exhibitions, the disadvantage of this type of poster is that it is cumbersome and therefore unsuited to transportation by air, or other means where space is limited and the risk of damage is high.

Card presentation. If travelling interstate or overseas the 'multi-card' system is an extremely convenient form of presentation. In this type of poster, each part of the research process is described and/or illustrated on A4 sized pieces of stiff card, which makes the poster both less likely to curl when displayed or to be damaged in transit. In addition the 'Multicard' system is extremely flexible as the cards can be added to or amended as the need arises, and may be prepared so as to fit into a brief case for easy transportation.

Choosing the right format

Before deciding upon which form your poster will take, you will need to ascertain the display conditions imposed by the conference organisers. These specifications will normally include recommendations as to size as well as the facilities available for the attaching the poster to the display fixtures. If fabric covered boards are available, consider using Velcro or similar material on the back of your poster or cards. Velcro is an extremely convenient and quick method of mounting a poster as it adheres readily to fabric covered boards. Unlike drawing pins it will not cause any damage with prolonged or repeated use. If only hard surfaces are available, consider using Blutack in preference to adhesive tape, which may damage the poster if its weight causes it to tear away from its mounting.

Designing your poster

The most successful posters are those which use photographs and/or other attractive graphics to illustrate the most important aspects of the study. In this regard, pages of typewritten text glued to a single sheet of thin card are to be *avoided* at all costs. When preparing your poster use words sparingly—

describe briefly the aim of the study, the research question, the methodology and data analysis. Any text included should be in upper and lower case letters and be large enough to be read from a distance of at least two metres.

If your study incorporated a change in practice, use photographs (at least 20 cm × 30 cm) to demonstrate the change, rather than large blocks of descriptive text. Wherever possible, illustrate your results using attractive figures, graphs and/or tables.

Organise the content of your poster in a logical order, and try to make it obvious where one should begin looking at it. Leave plenty of space between each part of the poster, and exclude any information which may distract the observer from the main point of the research. Finally, choose a brief but interesting title, which will attract attention, and, if your study has been published, include the reference of the article on the poster.

Presenting your poster

To allow people to get the most from poster sessions, you may be required to give a brief overview of your research to an audience. In practice this usually involves little more than reading your abstract, and with some rehearsal it should present no problems for even the most nervous presenter. During the designated poster sessions, you will need to be available to answer questions. At these times it is useful to have a brief summary of the research and the reprints of (or references to) papers arising from the study, which you can give to people who want more information. When you cannot be present in person to present your poster, leave a pile of handouts and a note pad and pencil near the display so that people can contact you for further information.

Conclusion

In reality, the means which you choose to disseminate your findings will depend on the extent of your skills in speaking and writing and the opportunities which present themselves immediately after the completion of your research.

Wherever new journals are seeking prospective contributors, or articles related to your specialty, or conference organisers are seeking speakers or posters on subjects related to your research, the opportunity exists for you to add to the knowledge base of nursing. While the key to the successful dissemination of findings is choosing the medium to present them which suits you best, the most important thing of all is to share the results of your research with other nurses. The guidelines outlined in this chapter have been used successfully in the past and should enable you to present the findings of your study in the most appropriate way.

REFERENCES

Day R A 1989 How to write and publish a scientific paper, 3rd edn. Cambridge University
    Press, Cambridge
Grimmond T 1992 How to deliver effective presentations. Effective Presentations,
    Blackwood SA
Hawkins C, Sorgi M 1985 Research: how to plan, speak and write about it. Springer-Verlag,
    New York ˙
Sheridan D R, Dowdney D L 1986 How to write and publish articles in nursing. Springer,
    New York
Tornquist E 1986 From proposal to publication: an informal guide to writing about nursing
    research. Addison Wesley, Menlo Park, California

Resources

BOOKS

Basic steps in planning nursing research from question to proposal, 3rd edn

P. J. Brink, M. J. Wood
Jones & Bartlett, Boston, 1988

This book deals solely with the planning of the research process, commencing with finding a research topic, and ending with the written proposal. It is a book well suited to the beginning researcher, as is evidenced by its consistent use of plain language.

The book works systematically through all the elements of the research process under the basic tenet that 'research is only as good as its plan, and that a well conceived plan is of immeasurable assistance throughout the rest of the process'. Well emphasised is the importance of writing a basic researchable question that will logically lead to the rest of the research plan. Following on from this is a succinct discussion on reviewing relevant literature; research design; data collection (including reliability and validity of research instruments); planning for data analysis; human rights; and the art of writing a proposal. A list of recommended readings to supplement the content is provided at the end of each chapter.

Six sample research proposals form the Appendix, a wise inclusion as students often need to see an example to conceptualise what is required. The sample proposals cover the three levels of research as expounded in the book: exploratory, descriptive and experimental, plus a methodological study.

Davina Poroch
Sir Charles Gairdner Hospital, WA

Directory of nursing research in Australia 1989–1991, and 1991–1993 (in preparation)

Royal College of Nursing, Australia

As the title suggests, this extremely useful directory provides an overview of research activity by nurses or about nursing. It includes brief descriptive entries of research in progress and/or completed since 1989. The comprehensive index lists projects by both subject and author, thus making the document extremely user friendly. It is an invaluable reference for nurses wishing to review Australian studies or network with other researchers with similar research interests.

Jeanette Robertson
Princess Margaret Hospital for Children, WA

Essentials of nursing research, 4th edn

L. Notter, J. Hott
Springer, New York, 1987

This is an excellent beginning nurse researcher's resource book, written by two experienced nurses with experience in education, administration, clinical nursing and research. The contents provide an introduction to research, including its evolution, meaning and purpose; the research process, including ethical considerations, theoretical frameworks, data collection techniques, probability theory and report writing; and evaluation of research including critical analysis of articles in terms of credibility and significance for practice. The authors provide a wealth of illustrations from clinical nursing research reports to amplify the text. The book also includes an annotated list of studies (some of which are discussed in detail), references, glossary and a detailed index.

Nadine Gibbons
Mt Henry Hospital, WA

Instruments for clinical nursing research

M. Frank-Stromborg, editor
Jones & Bartlett, Boston, 1992

Wherever there is clinical nursing research, there is a need for an appropriate instrument to measure the variable under investigation. This book provides a comprehensive overview of a selection of valid and reliable instruments which have been developed to measure various functional states and clinical problems. The first part of the book describes how to evaluate instruments for use in clinical nursing research. The second part gives a detailed account of instruments developed to assess health and function such as hope, body image, sleep and conscious state. The third part describes instruments which may be used to measure clinical problems such as pain, dyspnoea and skin integrity. It is recommended as a primary resource for all nurses seeking valid and reliable instruments to measure clinical phenomena.

Jeanette Robertson
Princess Margaret Hospital for Children, WA

Measurement in nursing research, 2nd edn

C. F. Waltz, O. L. Strickland, E. R. Lenz
FA Davis & Co, Philadelphia, 1991

This text, now in its second edition, is a valuable reference for those seeking to design and test, or select a data collection instrument suited to the measurement of variables relevant to nursing. Theories of measurement and instrument design are clearly presented, as is the application of validity and reliability concepts to norm and criterion referenced measures. Well chosen examples from the practice setting and the use of simple tables and figures enhance this book, which has been written with the needs of students in nursing programs, as well as those of experienced practitioners seeking to develop their research expertise, in mind.

Jeanette Robertson
Princess Margaret Hospital for Children, WA

Measurement of nursing outcomes, vols 1-4

O. Strickland, C. Waltz, editors
Springer, New York, 1988, 1990

This set of volumes has been compiled to disseminate information about the measurement of clinical and educational nursing outcomes. Compiled from the results of a workshop which focused on the development and testing of tools suitable for nursing research, each volume covers a specific subject area. In volumes 1 and 4 the topics covered relate to the measurement of client outcomes, self care and coping skills. Those tools suitable for the measurement of nursing performance, professional development and clinical skills are presented in volumes 2 and 3. Each of the tools described is accompanied by a comprehensive description of its origin and purpose. A summation of the content and a comprehensive reference list concludes each chapter. These books are a rich source of valid measurement instruments, which nurses seeking to study clinical or educational outcomes may well find extremely useful.

Jeanette Robertson
Princess Margaret Hospital for Children, WA

Nursing research: the application of qualitative approaches

P. A. Field, J. M. Morse
Chapman and Hall, London, 1992

Field and Morse have written an invaluable handbook for novice or experienced qualitative nurse researchers. This concise little book gives directions in all phases of the qualitative research process. Good use of examples of nursing studies has been made to illustrate the different methods of qualitative research and data collection. It is an extremely user friendly volume, enhanced by a realistic approach to some of the more complex aspects of the research process.

Elspeth Oliver
Sir Charles Gairdner Hospital, WA

Nursing research: mistakes and misconceptions

L. Hockey
Churchill Livingstone, Edinburgh, 1985

With refreshing honesty and a sense of humour, Hockey provides a very readable account of her 25 years research experience, 'to warn others of things that I would like to have been warned about myself.' Commencing with basic essentials, such as the significance of clearly defining the research question, this book deals with many essential facets of organising a research project. Useful hints are provided for searching relevant literature, designing questions for both interviews and questionnaires, accessing a study population and dealing with field work hazards. In addition, advice on basic research etiquette is given to promote maximum co-operation from all involved in the project. Personal experiences are shared throughout, allowing the reader to appreciate both how difficulties were encountered, and how they were addressed. Each chapter concludes with a summary of hindsight advice, with a further summary in the epilogue to reinforce the salient points made throughout the book. The book is recommended as an excellent handbook for the novice, and not-so-novice, nurse researcher.

Sue Tudor Owen
Sir Charles Gairdner Hospital, WA

Nursing research: principles and methods, 4th edn

D. F. Polit, B. P. Hungler
J.B. Lippincott, Philadelphia, 1991

Since the release of its first edition in 1978, this book has been regarded as a primary resource for nursing research. In the 4th edition, the previous logical, systematic treatment of each facet of the nursing research process has been retained, and the chapters on data collection and analysis expanded. New chapters on ethical considerations and the integration of qualitative and quantitative research methods enhance the new edition which includes many examples to illustrate various aspects of the nursing research process.

Jeanette Robertson
Princess Margaret Hospital for Children, WA

Paths to knowledge: innovative research methods for nursing

B. Sarter, editor
National League of Nursing, New York, 1988

This book contains some interesting material on nursing knowledge and types of qualitative research methodologies with application to nursing. Of the methods outlined, a good background for each is provided. As they are written by different authors however, they vary in focus and direction. For a researcher looking for specific information on how to apply qualitative methods, the chapters on ethnography, grounded theory, meta-analysis and esthetic inquiry are particularly useful. The chapter on future research is excellent, as are the chapters on ethical and philosophical aspects which are good for understanding the wider implications of knowledge. While not recommended for use in isolation, the contents of this book complement other research texts.

Anne Williams
Sir Charles Gairdner Hospital, WA

Research and statistics: a practical introduction for nurses

C. M. Hicks
Prentice Hall, New York, 1990

In explaining the basic concepts of research, this book provides the novice nurse researcher with a practical introduction to the elements of research design and the analysis of data in sixteen chapters, each of which concludes with a particularly valuable summary of the key points and glossary of key words and terms. In addition to worked examples of a variety of statistical tests, there are numerous opportunities throughout the text for readers to work through practical exercises. Answers to these problems are provided in the comprehensive Appendix, along with basic mathematical principles, symbols found in statistical formulae and statistical probability tables.

Overall this book is extremely useful. It provides a clear description of research methods and statistics and is recommended to all beginners about to undertake research.

Pat Mannion
(formerly) Royal Perth Hospital, WA

Research in nursing, 2nd edn

H. Wilson
Addison Wesley, Redwood City CA, 1989

This comprehensive text, written by an experienced nurse researcher and educator provides the nursing student with the basic knowledge and skills required to undertake an investigation. It also provides an informative resource reference for the more advanced researcher. The book is divided into four parts. Part 1 provides an introduction to the research process and its significance to patient care. Part 2 focuses on research skills, including the vocabulary for preparing a complete, formal critique. Part 3 includes a comprehensive overview of the research process, including qualitative and quantitative data collection techniques. A description of data analysis, statistical procedures and computer utilisation is also provided. Part 4 covers the specific guideline and strategies for communicating findings in documentary and oral presentations.

There is also an extensive glossary of research terminology, resources and samples in the appendix.

Nadine Gibbons
Mt Henry Hospital, WA

Research methods: principles, practice and theory for nursing, 3rd edn

C. Seaman
Appleton Lange, Norwalk, 1987

Originally written for undergraduate students, this book provides a useful overview of nursing research for the complete beginner. Divided into six parts, the chapters cover the fundamental elements and theory underlying the research process, in addition to the simple, but more than adequate, account of each aspect of the research process. Samples of questionnaires and observation forms are provided in the comprehensive Appendix, which also contains an extensive glossary. The strength of this book is the author's ability to provide a comprehensive coverage of the theory and practice of nursing research in an extremely user friendly form. It is particularly recommended for novice researchers, or as a resource for those having difficulty comprehending the methods or measurements described in more advanced texts.

Jeanette Robertson
Princess Margaret Hospital for Children, WA

Statistics for health professionals

S. Shott
W. B. Saunders Co., Philadelphia, 1990

This is an excellent text and reference book that provides readers with a good understanding of both univariate and multivariate statistical procedures. No degree of mathematical sophistication is required to use this book successfully. Its aim is to impart the assumptions necessary for selecting an appropriate test, rather than how to calculate specific formulae.

Emphasis is placed on the correct interpretation of statistical results produced by the SPSS and SAS software programs. Algorithms for selecting statistical procedures are provided, as are the answers to many of the problems discussed in the text.

The book is well organised and well written, and concentrates on the application and interpretation of statistical methods.

Sunita McGowan
Fremantle Hospital, WA

SOFTWARE

Epi-Info

Epi-Info is a public domain software package of integrated programs, which can both process epidemiological data, and organise study designs and results into a text format suitable for the production of written reports. The processing of data may be initiated through the production of a questionnaire in the word processing program. Alternatively data may be imported directly from pre-existing delimited, fixed length, dBase or SAS files. The analysis program is capable of performing a variety of statistical functions. Its output is characteristically lists, frequencies and cross tabulations, accompanied by inferential statistical calculations. Epi-Info can also be used as the basis of a surveillance system using a data base format. Data files are limited in size only by disc space. Graphics can also be generated by the program, which requires an IBM compatible PC with DOS, 512kb of RAM and at least one floppy disc drive.

Coralie Hill
Swan District Hospital, WA

Ethnograph

Ethnograph is designed to assist the ethnographic or qualitative researcher in those *mechanical* aspects of text data analysis which was traditionally handled using the cut-and-paste or card methods. Running the program results in the transcription or conversion of text data generated by word processing programs into a 40 column format in which each line of text numbered. By manually coding the lines or segments of text, data may be 'code mapped'. The 'nesting and overlapping' system enables a single line of text to be incorporated into a maximum of 12 different codes.

Once entered into the program, the contextual comments or reminders can be accommodated in the text to assist with the interpretation and analysis of the data. The 'search and locate' function groups coded lines or segments ready for printing. Single or multiple code searches can be facilitated by Ethnograph which greatly enhances the speed and accuracy of qualitative data analysis.

Coralie Hill
Swan District Hospital, WA

Excel

Microsoft Excel is a powerful spreadsheet capable of analysing and graphically representing quantitative data. In the worksheet format, Excel functions to manipulate, analyse and calculate data. Tables may also be created using pre-defined formats. Using the database function, data may be sorted and searched using standard operations. The graphics component of the program enables high quality graphs and charts to be generated directly from the worksheet and exported to word processing applications such as Word or Word Perfect. Conversely data may be imported directly from SAS, SPSS, Lotus or dBase III files.

Jeanette Robertson
Princess Margaret Hospital for Children, WA

NUDIST

If you are looking for a system to manage and organise qualitative data, and/or support its analysis, the 'Non-numerical Unstructured Data Indexing Searching and Theorising' or NUDIST software is worth considering. Typically the analysis of qualitative data requires the compilation and indexing (coding) of documents to be analysed, searching the printed text for key words and phrases, annotating the text with emerging themes and reminders and reorganising your indexing as your analysis progresses. These processes occur throughout the lifetime of the project and affect each other. The NUDIST system is unique in its support for all these procedures. It also contains many features found in no other qualitative software such as the ability to:

- index off-line documents;
- index documents under whatever categories you choose (subcategories are unlimited);
- change indexes easily;
- reorganise hierarchical categories;
- retrieve extracts of documents in various ways to express questions or hypotheses;
- build new categories from old;
- store text searches in an index; and
- store unlimited comments at any category to record thinking.

Tony Fetherston
Edith Cowan University, WA

Statistical Analysis System (SAS)

While SAS does not enjoy a reputation for being particularly user friendly, with a little practice, users will find SAS to be an extremely powerful system capable of a wide range of functions related to the management, analysis and presentation of data. The basic SAS system provides for:

- storage and retrieval of information;
- modification and processing of data;
- generation of reports and graphics; and
- calculation of descriptive statistics and summaries.

Extended applications of these operations may be achieved with the installation of additional optional programs designed to enhance the basic SAS functions of data analysis and management.

Jeanette Robertson
Princess Margaret Hospital for Children, WA

Standards

The following standards for nursing research were compiled in 1990 by members of the Western Australian Nurse Researchers' Network:

STANDARD 1

Nurses undertaking research will respect the basic human rights of the individual at all times

Criteria

1. Research which requires human subjects will show evidence of protection of the individual's right:

- not to be harassed
- to full disclosure
- to self determination
- to privacy, anonymity and confidentiality
- to refuse or withdraw from participation without the threat of reprisal as specified in the:
  - Nuremberg Code
  - Declaration of Helsinki
  - International Council of Nurses Statement
  - Australian Nursing Federation Policy Statement
  - National Health and Medical Research Council Statement on Ethics

2. Captive populations, e.g. children, the mentally or physically ill, the handicapped, students or prisoners should only be used where normal populations are unsuitable for the purposes of the study.

STANDARD 2

Research undertaken by nurses will utilise methodology appropriate for the study question

Criteria

1. Research proposals will address issues related to:
   1.1   reliability and validity
   1.2   adequacy of sample size

1.3   analytical plan
1.4   relationship of proposed research to established theory

2. Research reports will include relevant data (including any negative evidence obtained) and clearly state any limiting factors of the study.

3. Where the level of skill and knowledge required to complete a project extends beyond the expertise of the researcher, evidence of consultation with appropriate experienced personnel will exist.

STANDARD 3

Nurses undertaking research will seek to promote the concept of research in nursing and health

Criteria

1. Nurses undertaking research in organisations or agencies will:
    1.1   observe the philosophical foundation of the organisation/agency.
    1.2   seek membership on those committees which are relevant to job responsibilities, e.g.
        • Research and Ethics Committee
        • Nursing Research Committee
        • Patient Care Committee
        • Quality Improvement Committee
        • Nursing Standards Committee
        • Committees of Professional Organisations
    1.3   act as a consultant/resource to facilitate research.
    1.4   provide educational opportunities designed to inform and involve nurses in the research process.
    1.5   disseminate findings of research in appropriate forums and publications.

STANDARD 4

Nurses undertaking research will demonstrate efficient use of research resources

Criteria

1. Prepared budgets will reflect cost effective use of human and material resources.

2. Accurate records of income and expenditure will be maintained as requested.

3. Sources of support for nursing research will be actively pursued when appropriate.

4. Where appropriate, research grants will be sought from sources outside the organisation to supplement the costs of research activities.

STANDARD 5

Nurses undertaking research will actively seek to maintain and improve the quality of nursing research

Criteria

1. References to current professional literature will be evident in research protocols developed by nurses undertaking research.
2. Nurses undertaking research will seek to participate in education programs and conferences relevant to their needs and interests.
3. Nurses undertaking research will seek to foster communication with agencies where assistance for projects may be forthcoming.
4. The process of nursing research will be subjected to ongoing quality improvement monitoring.

Index

AARNet (Australian Academic
    and Research Network), 28
abstract, for research articles, 158
acceptance of research article pending
    modifications, 160-1
access to participants, for the study, 36
acknowledgments, 157
acutely ill subjects, collecting data from,
    112-13
ADONIS, 28
allocation of subjects to study groups, 55-6,
    86-8
    matching subjects, 87-8
    medical record numbers, 87
    random numbers, 87
analysing data, once collected, 43
analysis of qualitative data, 142-50
ANOVA, 131
application form, for grants, completion, 39,
    47
application procedures, for grants, 39
Applied Social Sciences Index and Abstracts,
    20
approaching patients, as subjects, 80-2
assessing the feasibility of a research setting,
    68
Australasian Medical Index, 23, 28
Australian Bibliographic Network (ABN),
    28
Australian Health Ethics Committee, 52
Australian Journal of Advanced Nursing, 19,
    22
Australian Nurses' Journal, 20
Australian Public Affairs Information
    Service (APAIS), 20
availability
    of equipment or consumable items, 69
    of research awards, 38
    of subjects, 68

background to the study, 40-2, 53
bar charts, 132, 133
bibliographic databases, 22-6
bibliographic formats, 22
bibliographies, 19, 20

blank spaces in a record, accounting for,
    125-6
blinding techniques, 56
books, on nursing research, 171-7
Boolean connectors, 24-5
budget, for the research proposal, 43-4

card presentation for posters, 168
case, definition, 119
CD-ROM databases, 5, 23
CD-ROM full text document storage, 28
children
    aspects of test administration, 93-4
    collecting data from, 92-3, 94
    modifying standardised tools for use by,
        93
    recruiting, 83-4
child's privacy, 83, 84
choosing a journal, to submit publications,
    152-3
choosing a valid data collection instrument,
    69-72
CINAHL, 17, 21, 152
citation indexes, 21
clarity in grant writing, 45-6
clinical nursing research
    definition, 1
    reasons for conducting, 2-3
clinical research
    implementation, 88-9
    ongoing management, 89-90
    pilot studies, 76-7
    planning summary, 117
    problems, 105-17
co-authorship, 12
coding, of qualitative data, 143
colleagues as subjects, recruiting, 79
collecting data, 43
    by interview, 90-2
    from children, 92-3
    from difficult subjects, 113-14
    from elderly subjects, 95-6
    from illiterate subjects, 113
    from special groups, 112-14
    from subjects who are acutely ill, 112-13

collecting data cont'd
    problems, 110-11
        compliance by staff, 110-11
        compliance by subjects, 111
    researcher's role, 89-90
    using questionnaires, 96-100
    see also data collection *headings*
column numbers, 123
command file, 120
completing the application form, 47
compliance by staff
    lack of expertise, 110-11
    requirements seen as a burden, 110
compliance by subjects, 111
    assessment, 111
computer software, 177-9
    for processing qualitative data, 142-3
computerisation, in the research study, 11
concepts, in research, 8
conditions for grants, 38-9
conduct of the study, influencing factors,
        68-9
conference presentations, 163-7
confidentiality, of information, 57, 79, 84,
        91, 103, 116
confirmatory matrices, 145, 146, 147, 149,
        150
consent
    from children, 83
    of all persons in study, 56-7, 80, 81
    to tape an interview, 91
consent forms, 56, 81
contact summary form, 139-40
content specialists, 72
control groups, and allocation of subjects,
        55-6
convenience sampling, 79
co-operation of other groups, in the
        research, 35
cultural differences, coping with, 116
*Cumulative Index to Nursing and Allied Health
        Literature see* CINAHL
current nursing practices, justification of,
        2-3

data analysis procedure, determination, 12
data checking, 125
data collection *see* collecting data
data collection forms, 11
data collection instruments, 69-72
    content, 72
    developing, 71-2
    format, for use by the elderly, 96
    modifying an existing instrument, 70-1
    modifying with children, 93
    modifying with elderly subjects, 95-6
    sensitivity, 98
    statistical advice, 72
    using a pre-existing instrument, 70

    validity and reliability, 72
data collection log, 138-9
data collection phase, researcher's role
        during, 89-90
data entry, 126
data file, 120
data file print-out, visual inspection, 126-7
data generation, 137
data management, 136
data preparation
    accounting for blank spaces in a record,
        125-6
    checking the data, 125
    data entry, 126
    data transformation, 127-9
    inspecting the data file print-out, 126-7
    recording errors, 126
    running frequency counts, 127
data processing, 129-31
data processing record, 137-8
data transformation, 127-9
database entries, 24
database management package, for
        bibliographic references, 27
database searching, 22-6
description of the proposed study, 40-3
descriptive research, pilot studies, 76
dictionaries, 17
difficult subjects, collecting data from,
        113-14
directional hypothesis, 9
directories, 17
discussion, in research articles, 157
disruption
    of the research setting, 108-9
    of the work force, 109
disseminating findings, 151-69
document record, 140
double blind studies, 56
drafts of research articles, 158-9

elderly subjects
    aspects of test administration, 96
    collecting data from, 956
    format of data collection instruments, 96
    modifying standard tools for use by, 85-6
    recruiting, 85-6
electronic delivery of library information, 28
electronic searching, 22-6
    advantages, 23
    strategy, 24-6
eligibility for research awards, 38
eligible subjects not approached, 106-7
empirical and theoretical information, 18
end-user search packages, 23
enlisting assistance, for the study, 11-12
enquiry letters to editors, 159
environmental temperature, as reason for
        replication studies, 6

Epi-Info (computer software), 177
equipment calibration, 88-9
ethical considerations
    and scientific integrity, 56
    in research proposals, 33, 35
ethics committees, 49-65
    and consent from all subjects, 56-7
    and misconduct in research, 59-60
    and securing approval for protocols,
        60-5
    and the research protocol, 52-6
    membership, 50-1
    presentation of protocol to, 63-5
    regulation of research, 51-2
    roles, functions and expectations of,
        49-60
    scrutiny of questionnaires, 58
    submission of protocol to, 58
Ethnograph (computer software), 138, 142,
    144, 177
Excel (computer software), 178
exploratory matrices, 145, 146, 147, 148
extra subjects in study, 86

feasibility of the study, 33, 34-5
feedback, on research outcome, 79
field, definition, 119
field size, 123
file, definition, 120
filing system, for qualitative studies, 142
filter questions, 97
    transforming, 129
financing your research project, 31-47, 54
frequency counts, for variables, 127
frequency distributions, 131
front-end search packages, 23
full text electronic document storage, 28
funding
    for the study, 11
    purpose of, 37-8
funding agencies
    choosing, 37-9
    expectations, 31-3

galley proofs, 162
grant application, compiling, 34-7
grant proposals, writing, 39-44
grants
    conditions for, 38-9
    writing style, 44-7
graphical presentation of data, 132-3
graphs, 130, 133
GRATIS library network, 27
grouping data, to extend the boundaries,
    127-8
guidelines (institutional)
    compliance with, 62
    for research, 61
guidelines on misconduct in research, 59-60

HealthROM, 28
histograms, 130, 132, 133
human experimentation, NH&MRC views,
    51-2
· hypothesis statement, in research articles,
    154-5

illiterate subjects, collecting data from, 113
implementing clinical research, 88-9
    calibration of equipment, 88
    preparing nursing staff, 88
incentives/rewards, for subjects of research,
    94, 104
Index Medicus, 20, 21, 23
inferential statistics, 130-1
    assumptions of normality, 131
    level of measurement, 131
information manager, use of, 19-20
information searching, 15-29
information sources, identification, 19
informativeness in grant writing, 44-5
informed consent see consent
institutional ethics committee meeting
        preparing for the meeting, 63-4
        presentation of research protocol, 63-5
        winning approval at the meeting, 64-5
Institutional Ethics Committees, 33, 35,
        49-52, 56-65, 68, 78, 80
institution's guidelines for research, 61
    compliance with, 62
insufficient patient focused research, 3
insufficient potential subjects, 106
inter-library loan services, 27
International Nursing Index (INI), 17, 20, 21,
        22, 23, 152
Internet system, 28
interpreters, 115
interrater reliability, establishing, 74-5, 77,
        109
interviews
    as method of collecting data, 90-2
    comfortable setting for, 116
    setting up appointments, 90-1
    with nurses in the work setting, 92
    with patients, 91-2
    with subjects at home, 91-2
introduction, in research articles, 154

journal abbreviations, 22
journal articles, 5
journal indexes, 20-2
journal style guides, 153-4, 159
journals
    choosing for place of publication, 152-3
    frequency of publication, 153
    place of publication, 152-3
    potential readership, 152
    refereed and non-refereed, 153
    style and emphasis, 152

knowledge base, 12
known experts, 19
known studies, 19

language differences, coping with, 114-15
length of record, 124
library catalogues, 20
library classification schemes, 27
library collections and services, 27-8
    costs involved, 28
    electronic delivery, 28
Likert scale, 98, 119, 121, 128
limitations to your own skills, 12
List of Lists, 78
literature review, 5, 41-2
    aim, 15-16, 26
    search planning, 16-18
    searching principles, 16
    writing the, 28-9
local area networks (LANs), 23
logical operators, 24-5
loss of research setting, 108-9

mailing lists, 78
master sheet, 140-1
matching questionnaires, strategies, 101-2
matching subjects, 87-8
matrix analysis, 144-50
medical record numbers, as basis for
    randomisation, 87
Medical Subject Headings (MeSH), 17, 158
Medline, 23
mentally impaired subjects, recruiting, 84-5
methodology, appropriateness of, 32
misconduct in research, 59-60
multiple response questions, 124, 125
Mystat (statistical package), 119, 128

National Health and Medical Research
    Council
    ethics committee composition, 50
    Statement on Human Experimentation,
        51-2
networking, 19
NH&MRC *see* National Health and Medical
    Research Council
non-directional hypothesis, 9
non-English speaking subjects
    coping with, 114-15
    documentation, 115
non-invasive interventions, 2, 3
non-parametric tests, 131
non-refereed journals, 153
    review process, 160
NUDIST (computer software), 142, 178
null hypothesis, 9
numerical data, presentation, 132-3
nurses as subjects, recruiting, 78-9
nurses not work colleagues as subjects,
    recruiting, 79-80

nursing journals, choosing for place of
    publication, 152-3
nursing literature, organisation, 18
nursing procedures, unvalidated, as research
    topics, 5
nursing research standards, 181-5
nursing specialisation, 2

objectives for the study, 41, 52-3
obtaining institution's guidelines for
    research, 61
obtaining university approval to commence
    your study, 61-2
omission of persons from study, reasons for,
    114
online databases, 23
oral presentations
    at seminars and conferences, 163-7
    preparation of visual aids, 164-5
    preparing the content, 163-4
    presenting your talk, 166-7
    rehearsing your talk, 165-6
    taking questions, 167
organising your retrieved records, 26-7
output file, 120
overhead projection films, 164-5, 166

parametric statistical tests, 131
parental consent, 83
patient interviews
    confidentiality, 91
    privacy, 91
    taping, 91
patients as subjects, recruiting, 80-3
patient's rights in research, 80, 81
Pearson's product moment correlation, 131
permission, for circulars to staff, 11
personal questions, 116-17
persuasiveness in grant writing, 46-7
photographs, in posters, 169
pie charts, 130, 132, 133
pilot studies, 75-8
    clinical research, 76-7
    descriptive research, 76
    evaluation, 77-8
placebo, 56
planning and conducting research, 67-104
planning your literature search, 16-18
poster presentations, 167-9
posters
    choosing the right format, 168
    design, 168-9
    presenting, 169
    types of, 168
practicalities of conducting the research, 10
pre- and post-intervention surveys, 101-2
preparation of visual aids, 164-5
preparing to collect data, 42-3
prerequisites of a proposal, 9-12
presentation of the research proposal, 33
presenting and reporting data, 43

presenting your research findings as a poster, 167-9
presenting your talk, 166-7
primary sources *vs* secondary sources, 18
printed indexes, 20-2
privacy, 83, 84, 91
problem definition, 6-8
problems
    conversion into a researchable format, 8-9
    in the clinical research setting, 105-17
procedure manuals, 5
professional responsibility, 3
profiling study participants, 129-30
progressing the analysis, of qualitative data, 144
project title, 40
proof reading
    of questionnaires, 100
    of research articles, 162
proposed research, descriptive plan of, 40-3
protocol *see* research protocol
psychiatric patients as subjects, recruiting, 84-5
Psychological Abstracts, 20
purpose of the funding, 37-8
purpose of the research, 40-1

qualitative data
    analysis, 142-50
    becoming familiar with the data, 143
    management, 135-50
qualitative methodologies, 8-9
qualitative research
    acceptance of by funding agencies, 38
    literature review, 16
quality assurance studies, 6
quantitative data, management, 119-34
quantitative methodologies, 9
quantitative research
    acceptance of by funding agencies, 38
    literature review, 15
questionnaires, 58
    commercial carrier distribution, 103-4
    confidentiality, 116
    covering letter, 99, 101-2
    design, 120-4
        formatting for computer analysis, 123-4
        order of questions, 122
        putting the question, 121-2
        using a diagram to put the question, 97, 123
    distributing to staff, 102
    for use with the elderly, 96
    instructions to respondents, 97-8
    matching, strategies, 101-2
    maximising distribution by staff, 102-3
    modification, 77
    optimising data collection with, 96-100
    optimising return rates by patients, 103
    preparation for printing, 99-100
    printing considerations, 100-1
    proof reading, 100
    returning, 99
    scaled responses, 98, 121-2
    sensitivity of instrument, 98, 122
    style and design, 100-1
    supplementary information, 98-9
    uninspiring, 112

random numbers, 87
rationale for conducting the research, 8, 41
recoding data, 128-9
record, definition, 120
record of contact form, 136
recording errors, 126
recording your progress, with qualitative data, 144
recruiting
    children as subjects, 83-4
    colleagues as subjects, 79
    elderly patients, 85-6
    nurses as subjects, 78-9
    nurses not work colleagues, 79-80
    patients as subjects
        approaching patients, 80-2
        preparation, 80
        withholding information, 82-3
    study subjects, 78-88
    subjects who are mentally impaired, 84-5
recruitment
    difficulties, 105-8
    eligible subjects not approached, 106-7
    insufficient potential subjects, 106
    slowness of, 105-6
recruitment of subjects, 54-5
    criteria, 55
    numbers to be recruited, 55
refereed journals, 153
    review process, 160-2
refining the search topic, 16-17
rehearsing your talk, 165-6
reject letters, types of rejection, 161-2
relevance of research, to funding agency, 31-2
relevance of the problem to the research setting, 67-8
relevance of the topic to practice, 9-10
replication studies, need for, 6
research articles
    abstract, 159
    accepted pending modifications, 160-2
    acknowledgments, 158
    description of the research methodology, 155-6
    discussion, 157
    format, 154-9
    introduction, 154
    reject letters, 161-2

research articles, cont'd
  reporting your results, 156-7
  review process, 160-2
  statement of the research question or
    hypothesis, 154-5
  submission to journal, 159-60
  title, 158-9
research assistants, 73-5
  interrater reliability, 74-5
  recruiting, 73-4
research awards
  eligibility and availability, 38
  value of, 38
research methodology, in research articles,
  155-6
research plan, 42-3
research project
  financing, 31-47
  implications for medical or allied health
    staff, 12
research proposal
  clarifying your thoughts, 34
  significance, 32
research protocol
  and ethics, 52
  and presentation at institutional ethics
    committee meetings, 63-5
  and scientific integrity, 56
  background information and scientific
    references, 53
  compliance with institution guidelines,
    62
  consent and confidentiality, 56-7
  control groups and allocation of subjects,
    55-6
  financial matters, 54
  objectives of the research, 52-3
  obtaining the institution's guidelines, 61
  obtaining the university approval to
    commence the study, 61-2
  practical strategies to secure approval,
    60-5
  recruitment of subjects, 54-5
  researchers involved, 56
  review of the documentation, 62-3
  study endpoints, 53-4
  submission, 58-9
    content, 58-9
  visit the proposed setting, 61
research question statement, in research
  articles, 154-5
research questions
  defining, 9
  on current practices, 2-3
research topic
  examples, 4-5
  selection, 3-6
  where to look, 5-6

researchable problems
  characteristics, 6-8
    nurses able to implement proposed
      changes, 7-8
    problem frequency in population, 6-7
    proposed solutions will improve
      patient care, 7
    unsatisfactory method of addressing
      current problem, 7
    valid and reliable way of
      measurement, 7
researchers, involved in project, 56
researcher's ability, 32
researcher's profile, 39-40
researcher's role, during data collection
  phase, 89-90
resource assessment, for the study, 33, 36-7
resources, for reference, 171-9
restrictions on access to subjects, 68-9
results section, in research articles, 156-7
retention of subjects, 107-8
review process, for submitted research
  articles, 160-2
reviewers, approach to nurse funding
  proposals, 31-3
rewards/incentives, for subjects of research,
  94, 104

scale, definition, 120
scientific integrity, and ethical
  considerations, 56
search planning, defining the scope of the
  search, 17-18
search topic, refining, 16-17
searching for information, 15-29
  principles, 16
searching the literature, 19-26
secondary sources vs primary sources, 18
selecting a research setting, 67
selecting a research topic, 3-6
selection of relevant articles, 26
seminar presentations, 163-7
sensitive topics, 116-17
significance of the project, 42
single blind studies, 56
single sheet posters, 168
slides, 165, 166
slow recruitment, 105-6
social differences, coping with, 116
Spearman's rank order correlation, 131
sponsors of nursing research, expectations,
  31-3
SPSS (Statistical Packages for the Social
  Sciences), 119, 127, 128, 129
staff changes, impact on data collection, 109
staff role, in recruitment of subjects, 106-7
staff skills, to collect data, 110-11
staff work load, impact of research project
  on, 69

standards, for nursing research, 181-5
statistical analysis, 130-1
Statistical Analysis System (SAS), 119, 178-9
statistical software packages, 110, 178-9
study endpoints, 53-4
style guides, 153-4, 159
subjects of research
    consent and confidentiality, 56-7
    incentives/rewards, 94, 104
    recruiting, 78-82
submitting your article, 159-60
succinctness in grant writing, 47
support infrastructure for the study
    personnel, 10
    physical resources, 10-11

t-tests, 131
tables, value of, 132
taking questions, at oral presentations, 167
talk content
    body of the talk, 164
    conclusion, 164
    formatting your notes, 164
    introduction, 163
talks
    at seminars and conferences, 163-7
    presentation, 166-7
    rehearsal, 165-6
taped interviews, transcribing, 137
taping an interview, 91
theoretical frameworks, 8
theoretical information, 18
thesauruses, 17

time frame, for the study, 10
title, of research articles, 158-9
toddlers, working with, 93
training sessions, for staff, 11-12
transcribing taped interviews, 137
typography, in printed questionnaires, 99-100

uniform during recruitment, 82
university approval to commence the study, 61-2
University of Western Australia, guidelines on misconduct in research, 59-60

values, definition, 120
variable, definition, 120
visit the proposed setting, 61, 68
visual aids, preparation, 164-5
Visual Analogue Scale, 97, 123
visual presentation of the proposal, 46

Western Australian Nurse Researchers' Network, standards, 181-5
withdrawal of subjects from clinical studies, 57, 108
withholding information, 82-3
word processing package, for bibliographic references, 27
work force disruption, impact on data collection, 109
writing
    for publication, 151-2
    grant proposals, 39-44
    the literature review, 28-9
writing style for grants, 44-7